Hip Replacement

Orthopedic Patient Education

Adam E. M. Eltorai, PhD, and
Alan H. Daniels, MD, Series Editors

Hip
Replacement

EXPERTS ANSWER YOUR QUESTIONS

Edited by

Adam E. M. Eltorai, PhD

Alan H. Daniels, MD

Derek R. Jenkins, MD

Lee E. Rubin, MD

JOHNS HOPKINS UNIVERSITY PRESS

Baltimore

© 2019 Johns Hopkins University Press
All rights reserved. Published 2019
Printed in the United States of America on acid-free paper
9 8 7 6 5 4 3 2

Johns Hopkins University Press
2715 North Charles Street
Baltimore, Maryland 21218-4363
www.press.jhu.edu

Library of Congress Cataloging-in-Publication Data

Names: Eltorai, Adam E. M., editor.
Title: Hip replacement : experts answer your questions / edited by
    Adam E. M. Eltorai, PhD, Alan H. Daniels, MD, Derek R. Jenkins, MD,
    and Lee E. Rubin, MD.
Description: Baltimore : Johns Hopkins University Press, 2019. | Series:
    Orthopedic patient education | A Johns Hopkins Press Health Book |
    Includes index.
Identifiers: LCCN 2018039698 | ISBN 9781421429571 (hardcover :
    alk. paper) | ISBN 1421429578 (hardcover : alk. paper) | ISBN
    9781421429588 (pbk. : alk. paper) | ISBN 1421429586 (pbk. : alk.
    paper) | ISBN 9781421429595 (electronic) | ISBN 1421429594
    (electronic)
Subjects: LCSH: Total hip replacement—Surgery—Popular works. |
    Hip joint—Surgery—Popular works.
Classification: LCC RD549 .H56 2019 | DDC 617.5/810592—dc23
LC record available at https://lccn.loc.gov/2018039698

A catalog record for this book is available from the British Library.

*Special discounts are available for bulk purchases of this book. For more
information, please contact Special Sales at specialsales@press.jhu.edu.*

CONTENTS

Every day in our medical offices, patients and their families ask great questions, eager to learn more about their hip condition. Patients want to know more about their symptoms, diagnoses, alternatives to surgery, when surgery is necessary, preparation for surgery, and recovery from surgery. Much of the currently available health information can be hard to access or comes from sources of dubious quality. There is a need for a practical, evidence-based source of information tailored specifically for the patient.

With elective surgery, patients are interested in gathering information to help choose the best course of treatment for themselves or their family members. This book is intended to serve as a complete guide for patients. The focus is on the patient experience, outlining the process, and anticipating and answering commonly asked questions. We include patient stories to help familiarize the experience of having hip pain, getting a diagnosis, and deciding on treatment. We use examples to explain everything patients want to know about their condition and all the available management options in order to help them determine the right treatment path for them.

The goal of this book is to make complex information accessible to our patients. We hope that this book serves as a resource that individuals can use when they have questions. Moreover, we hope that this book quells some of the natural anxieties and fears that patients might have when considering a hip replacement.

The book is organized into five chapters. The first chapter provides readers with a basic introduction to arthritis of the hip. In this chapter, you learn about arthritis, hip anatomy, and symptoms of hip arthritis. Additionally, we explain what you should prepare prior to your visit to your doctor. In chapter 2, you learn about alternatives to surgery, including lifestyle changes, medications, and surgical treatments other than hip replacement. We walk you through the factors to consider when deciding on surgery and the steps you will need to take to get medically cleared prior to surgery. Chapter 3 takes you through the various ways to prepare for a hip replacement, including both home preparation and self preparation. In chapter 4, we outline in detail a patient's time in the hospital, from registration to discharge. Finally, in chapter 5 we explain care after you leave the hospital. This chapter covers topics such as pain management, diet, and rehabilitation protocols. We hope that this book helps you to make the decision of whether to get a total hip replacement and, if you decide to go ahead with the surgery, that it will explain clearly what to expect from the surgery and recovery.

Hip Replacement

CHAPTER 1

Overview of Hip Arthritis

**Dominic T. Kleinhenz, MD, and
Valentin Antoci, Jr., MD, PhD**

Hip arthritis is "wear and tear" of the hip joint that occurs over time. Knowing the anatomy of the hip joint and hip arthritis can help you better understand why your hip arthritis hurts and how a hip replacement can help you. There are multiple causes of hip arthritis, which are explained in this chapter. People with hip arthritis usually see a doctor for hip pain, stiffness, or a combination of pain and stiffness. They may also see a doctor because they have lost the capacity to walk, to use stairs, or to do things that are required for basic daily activities and quality of life.

We will go through the ways that the surgeon evaluates you prior to hip replacement surgery. At the initial visit with your orthopedic surgeon, the doctor will work to confirm that hip arthritis is in fact the source of your hip pain. Before going forward with hip replacement surgery, you need to try nonsurgical strategies to manage your pain and stiffness. Anti-inflammatory medication, physical therapy, injections, and use of a cane or walker may provide enough relief to prevent surgery altogether. Your surgeon will talk to you about prior medical conditions, medications, surgeries, and allergies to get a better understanding of your health so your surgery will be as safe as possible.

What Is Arthritis?

Arthritis is not a single disease. It is a term used to refer to wear and tear of our joints over time, which causes damage to the normally smooth, slippery covering of the joint (cartilage). There are three main types of arthritis: osteoarthritis (OA), inflammatory arthritis, such as rheumatoid arthritis (RA), and post-traumatic arthritis. OA is the most common type of arthritis and occurs slowly over time due to repetitive stress on the joint. OA can affect any joint and leads to erosion of the protective cartilage. This in turn may lead to rough-ening of the surface, increased friction, bone-on-bone contact, growth of new bone (known as osteophytes

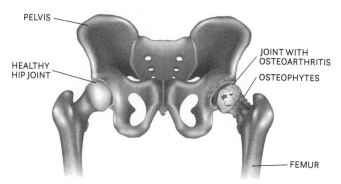

FIGURE 1.1. Hip joint osteoarthritis: a healthy hip joint compared to a joint with osteoarthritis

The amount of hip arthritis seen on your X-rays does not necessarily correlate to the amount of pain you are having. Two patients with the same hip X-rays may have different pain levels and different responses to nonsurgical treatment. Doctors like to say that they "operate on patients, not X-rays." If your X-rays show "bone on bone" arthritis but you are already getting good pain relief with anti-inflammatory medications, physical therapy, or using a cane or walker, it may not be a good time for surgery. But even if you don't have bone-on-bone arthritis, if you are no longer getting pain relief from things that previously helped, it may be time to go forward with surgery.

or bone spurs), and even loose pieces of bone or tissue floating in the joint, making pain worse or causing mechanical locking, clicking, or catching. Because OA is typically the result of damage over time, it mostly affects patients age 40 and older. However, certain people are genetically predisposed to OA and may develop it at an earlier age.

Diseases that affect joints are called arthropathies. Inflammatory arthropathies, such as RA, are caused by autoimmune disorders in which the body's own immune system attacks joints, causing them to deteriorate. It typically involves multiple joints. In addition to affecting the cartilage, autoimmune diseases cause overgrowth of the lining of the joint, the synovium, which contributes to additional pain and swelling. RA is a systemic disease that affects the whole body. It will typically involve the medical care of a rheumatologist, who will prescribe and manage powerful medications, in addition to surgical care from an orthopedist.

Lastly, post-traumatic arthritis occurs when degenerative changes of the joint result from an injury or trauma that leads to accelerated damage of the joint. This damage may be from fractured bone surfaces, disrupted blood supply, misalignment, an improperly healed fracture, cartilage injury, orthopedic hardware, infection, or a host of other causes. Soft tissue injuries in the hip, such as cartilage tears due to the ball-shaped head of the femur rubbing against the hip joint socket as a child or adolescent, can also alter normal hip mechanics and contribute to post-traumatic arthritis.

Symptoms

Hip arthritis refers to a loss of cartilage within the hip joint. As the weight-bearing surface wears, the movement is no longer as smooth, thus irritating the joint and surrounding tissues as well as making muscles move abnormally. It ultimately leads to complete degradation of the joint, and often a total hip arthroplasty (or hip joint replacement) is needed to restore motion and relieve this joint pain. Though this chapter focuses mainly on the basics of OA, the chapters following describe hip replacement and recovery and are relevant to all people who are considering hip replacement.

With hip osteoarthritis, certain symptoms are common.

- Pain and stiffness are the main symptoms of hip osteoarthritis. Typical pain associated with hip arthritis is usually felt in the groin, sometimes in the buttock, and rarely on the side.

- The arthritis pain can start as either sharp or dull, achy pain and usually becomes constant over time.

- People with hip arthritis may have difficulty climbing stairs, rising from a seated position, bending to put on socks and tie shoes, clipping toenails, or sitting down into a low car. Pain or weakness of the hip muscles causes a limp.

Pain and stiffness are the main symptoms of hip OA. Commonly, when asked to describe where our hips are located, we point to our sides at our waistband. Anatomically, however, the center of the hip joint is located right over the groin. As such, typical pain associated with hip arthritis is usually felt in the groin, sometimes in the buttock, and rarely on the side. One of the classic signs of arthritis is that stiffness occurs after prolonged periods of sitting or lying but often improves with movement or activity. In fact, pain on the side is typically a sign of inflammation of the fluid-filled sac (called a bursa) near the hip, which is known as greater trochanteric bursitis rather than hip arthritis.

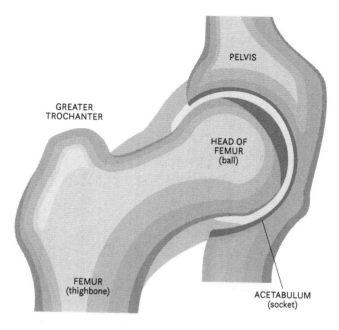

FIGURE 1.2. Hip anatomy (*side view*)

Arthritis pain can start as either a sharp or a dull, achy pain and usually becomes constant over time. It's almost like an asphalt road, which as it wears develops potholes that initially can be sharp and catching. As the road degrades further, the entire ride becomes uncomfortable, with more friction on the wheels. Arthritis pain typically worsens over months to years, even though the timeline is very unpredictable.

You might ask how long it will take until all the cartilage is gone and you may need a total hip replacement. The answer is unknown, as the disease progresses differently for each person. Sometimes, pain occurs suddenly after a fall or strenuous exercise. Stiffness is usually worst in the morning or after a period of rest and improves with activity, only to get even worse afterward or at the end of the day. People with hip arthritis may have difficulty climbing stairs, rising from a seated position, bending to put on socks and tie shoes, clipping toenails, or lowering themselves down into a car. Pain or weakness of the hip muscles causes a limp. Ultimately, having a hip replacement is like driving on a newly paved, ultrasmooth road. There is less friction, a quiet ride, and smooth driving once again.

Many people with hip arthritis experience a loss of range of motion or decreased flexibility. Some individuals with arthritis develop contractures. A contracture means that muscles and bone anatomy have changed to the point that the hip joint is stuck in one position. Most commonly, people are not able to turn the hip in or extend it all the way and end up with a leg that is slightly bent and rotated to the outside. This changes the normal way we walk, causing a limp, and may lead to hip bursitis and back pain. Quite commonly, people with hip pain also have back pain, and the opposite is also true. A cane, used in the hand opposite the pain, can improve the limp and help to decrease associated back pain or pain on the outside of the hip due to bursitis. There are many nonsurgical options for hip arthritis, which are discussed in chapter 2.

Hip Anatomy

The hip is a ball-and-socket joint formed by two bones. The bone of the hip socket is called the acetabulum and is physically connected to the pelvis bones. The top end of the femur, or thighbone, forms the ball. This joint is easy to visualize. It is similar in size to the trailer hitch and ball on a car or truck. To help the two surfaces glide by each other, both the acetabulum and the femur are covered in smooth, slippery cartilage. The joint space also contains a special lubricant called synovial fluid that helps the hip joint glide and allows the cartilage on the two bones to move smoothly on each other.

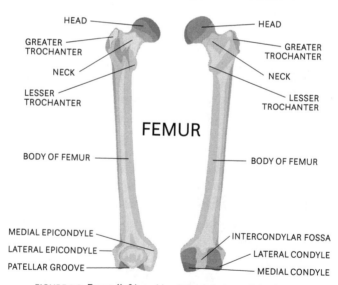

FIGURE 1.3. Front (*left*) and back (*right*) view of the femur

Anyone can develop hip OA, and the disease progression likely has a strong genetic component. Certain anatomical differences or previous trauma may distort the bony anatomy and normal mechanics, causing early wear and increasing the likelihood of developing arthritis. Most of these conditions lead to a mismatch between the ball and socket. Thus, the acetabulum or femur is not shaped correctly, and the abnormal movement causes arthritis. It's like trying to put a square peg in a round hole: they don't fit together.

- Anyone can develop hip OA, but the disease progression likely has a strong genetic component.
- Certain anatomical differences may make one more likely to develop hip arthritis.

OA starts with damage to the cartilage lining of the femur (ball) or the acetabulum (socket). When the cartilage wears away, the surface is no longer as smooth, and bits of cartilage and tissue can float around the joint almost like gravel, causing irritation called "synovitis." As the cartilage disappears, the bone that is exposed on the surfaces of the femur and acetabulum grind on each other. There is less joint space for the joint fluid, and the areas with remaining cartilage do not glide as smoothly. This is often referred to as "bone-on-bone" arthritis. The grinding of bones on each other causes pain. As the bone surfaces move on one another, the bones harden, a process called sclerosis.

Extra bone, called osteophytes or bone spurs, grows from the edges of the arthritic hip. When the spurs become large enough, they block movement and cause stiffness, pain, and mechanical sounds. As the anatomy gets more and more distorted, the symptoms typically get worse.

In a hip replacement surgery, the worn-out ball and socket of the arthritic hip joint is replaced with a new ball and socket. Most commonly the replacement ball, the femoral head, is metal or ceramic. A metal implant is placed in the top of the femur to hold the ball in place. The socket is replaced with a new metal, ceramic, or combination metal socket with plastic liner. Each of these types of hip replacements has its own risks and benefits. Be sure to ask your doctor what type of implant will be used in your surgery.

Diagnosis

Your doctor will make the diagnosis of hip arthritis based on your symptoms, history, physical exam, and imaging studies. Part of the work-up for arthritis will include X-rays. Your doctor orders X-rays of your pelvis and the painful hip to look for the abnormal anatomy and features of arthritis. More advanced imaging is typically not needed, as magnetic resonance imaging (MRI) does not usually provide useful additional information.

Your surgeon should treat you as an individual and **not an X-ray.** Imaging does not always correlate with symptoms—so even if you have bad-looking arthritis on X-ray, there is no need for a total hip arthroplasty if you are doing quite well and do not have much pain.

History

Patients' descriptions of their hip pain and symptoms are important for helping doctors understand their disease. Before even considering a total hip arthroplasty, nonsurgical strategies to manage the pain and stiffness should be tried. These include weight loss, nonsteroidal anti-inflammatory drugs (NSAIDs), steroid injections, physical therapy, and cane or walker use. Not all nonsurgical options work for everyone, and a complete story helps the doctor understand that. You should be prepared to answer the following:

- What brings you to the doctor? What hurts?
- What caused things to start hurting? Can you think of a specific event that may have been a factor?

- How long have you had these symptoms? When did they start?

- Where does it hurt precisely? Try to point to one spot.

- What makes symptoms worse? What makes symptoms better?

- Does your pain radiate—for instance, does the pain go down your legs?

- Have you had related symptoms or similar symptoms in the past?

Be sure that you try nonsurgical options to manage your hip arthritis before making the decision to have hip replacement surgery. Some patients can get many years of pain relief out of weight loss, physical therapy, injections, and cane or walker use. Not all patients have the same response to nonsurgical treatments. How much pain relief you will get from these nonsurgical options is hard to predict. If these nonsurgical options once worked for you but don't anymore, it may be time to have hip replacement surgery.

Medical History

The patient's complete medical history, including what medications he or she takes, is very important. Any heart, kidney, liver, or lung problems may need further

Making sure that you are as healthy as possible can help prevent some complications after hip replacement surgery. Much of the evaluation before surgery is geared toward reducing your chance of infection after surgery. You should have a dental checkup prior to surgery, ensuring that there is no infection in your teeth. If you have diabetes, keeping your blood sugar under control is very important in reducing risk of infection after surgery. Talk to your primary care doctor if you think you can improve your blood sugar control before surgery. After surgery, ask your doctor if you need antibiotics before having any other surgeries or dental procedures.

testing before surgery. Diabetes is an important part of the medical history because a poorly controlled blood sugar level can increase the risk of infection and cause trouble healing after surgery. An up-to-date hemoglobin A1C (three-month blood sugar measurement) helps show good glucose control. Your doctor can order this blood test. People who bruise easily or have frequent nose bleeds, heavy menstrual periods, bleeding gums, or family members with these problems may have a blood clotting problem that needs to be addressed before surgery. People who have had prior blood clots in the legs or lungs may need additional protection from blood clots after surgery. People with anemia, or low red blood cell counts, should be informed about the risk of blood loss from surgery and possible need for blood transfusion afterward. A personal or religious objection to blood transfusion may require additional planning before surgery. Regular dental visits and good dental habits before surgery can help reduce the risk of infection. Any dental visits after surgery should be discussed with your surgeon. Urinary tract infections or skin problems around the problem hip, legs, or feet in the weeks leading up to surgery should also be brought to the attention of the surgeon.

Medications

Medications that can potentially increase the risk of bleeding from surgery may be temporarily stopped or continued at a different dose prior to surgery. These medications include blood thinners, such as aspirin, warfarin (Coumadin), clopidogrel (Plavix), apixaban (Eliquis), rivaroxaban (Xarelto), and enoxaparin (Lovenox), and NSAIDs, such as ibuprofen (Advil, Motrin) and naproxen (Naprosyn). When to stop these medications and restart after the surgery is determined prior to surgery with the help of the patient's primary care provider and cardiologist, if they have one. Aspirin is now often being continued up to and after surgery without stopping or restarted soon afterward. Taking pain medications, especially narcotic pain medications, for a period of time before surgery can make pain control with additional medication more difficult after surgery. It is recommended to try to decrease the need for narcotic pain medication prior to surgery.

This should be done safely, under a doctor's supervision, as sudden decreases in pain medication can cause withdrawal symptoms. Steroids, especially when used over time, can decrease the amount of natural steroids that your body produces. If steroids cannot be stopped prior to surgery, a higher dose of steroids, called a "stress dose," may be needed on the day of surgery. Whether to stop taking medications before and after surgery will be discussed in chapters 3 and 4.

Any surgery, especially hip replacement surgery, can increase your risk of blood clots in the legs. The problem with blood clots in the legs is that they can travel to the lungs and cause difficulty breathing or put stress on your heart. Because of the risk of blood clots, your surgeon will start you on a blood thinner after surgery. It is important to ask your doctor what blood thinner they plan on using after surgery. There are many different types of blood thinners. The foods you eat can affect how warfarin (Coumadin) works. If you are started on warfarin (Coumadin) after surgery, ask your doctor what foods to avoid.

Physical Exam

The medical history is an important part of the doctor-patient interaction, allowing the physician to understand the person's pain, and the physical exam is equally important in understanding the individual's functional limitations. The physical exam will probably include an assessment of limb alignment, that is, whether the person's legs are straight, "bow-legged," or "knock-kneed." A good physical exam can also determine whether one leg is longer than the other, though whether the patient *feels* that one leg is longer than the other may be quite different from what is the case in reality. Spine deformity, hip pathology, and developmental limb differences may contribute to changes in leg length independent of the hip.

The physical exam includes an attempt to locate the person's area of pain, usually the groin or thigh in someone with hip arthritis. In some cases, the exam also seeks to reproduce the individual's symptoms as well. The doctor examines the hip range of motion, or movement. The lower back and knees may be examined to make sure that those are not additional sources of pain. The muscles, nerves, and blood vessels in the entire leg are also examined for any problems that may also cause hip complaints.

Surgical History

Any prior surgery on the hip and leg may affect the plan during surgery. An individual's other surgical history may reveal more about his or her medical conditions. It is also important to know if there were any problems with the past surgeries. For example, did the person have a reaction to anesthesia? Were they nauseated after prior surgeries?

Family History

Learning about a family history of arthritis can be important for the doctor in predicting how other joints might be impacted by arthritis. Other associated risks should be carefully explored. For instance, knowing about a family history of malignant hyperthermia is critical for the anesthesiologist. Malignant hyperthermia is a very rare condition that can cause a rapid increase in body temperature and muscle contractions when a person receives general anesthesia.

> This is the time to explore your support system and let your family and friends know that you may need their help.

Social History

The social history helps the doctor with planning the recovery from surgery. An understanding of who lives with the patient and the makeup of the home can help predict whether the home will be a safe place to return to when leaving the hospital. It may be difficult for someone who lives alone or someone who lives on the upper floor of an apartment building to return home immediately after surgery. This is the time to explore your support system and let your family and friends know that you may need their help. Even though most people are able to walk around with a walker or cane after a surgery, obtaining help with shopping, cleaning, or cooking will make things much easier and decrease the chance for falls or injury when attempting to do too much too soon after surgery.

If you live alone or have multiple stairs in your home, it may be difficult for you to return home safely when you leave the hospital after surgery. Before surgery, your surgeon can help you decide whether you will need to go to a rehabilitation hospital or a skilled nursing facility when you leave the hospital. But it is difficult to know whether you will be able to go home until you have worked with the therapists. Physical therapists provide the surgeon with their recommendations. Certain types of insurance require you to stay in the hospital a certain number of nights before going to rehab or a nursing home.

Other parts of the social history include exercise habits, smoking, drugs, and alcohol use. Use of street drugs and tobacco are very important bits of information. Cocaine use around the time of surgery may increase the chance of a heart attack. Tobacco use is linked to poor wound healing and possible infection. Unfortunately, an infection in the hip may lead to significant disability. Quitting smoking improves the chances of successful surgery. In early arthritis, it may even slow down the progression of disease and loss of cartilage. Also, stopping smoking as little as two weeks before surgery can lower the risk of lung problems around the time of surgery.

Quitting smoking prior to surgery is not only good for your general health but can help you recover more easily after surgery. Quitting smoking as little as two weeks before surgery lowers the risk of lung problems after surgery. Smoking after surgery reduces blood flow to your incision and can make your incision slow to heal. Any problems with wound healing can lead to infection. Quitting smoking improves the health of your heart and lungs, which can help you walk longer distances without tiring and get more out of physical therapy. Vapor, e-cigarettes, chewing tobacco, and any other nicotine products also increase your risks.

Tests

Besides the clinical history and exam, X-rays are the main test used to diagnose hip arthritis. X-rays are painless images that use small doses of radiation to make a picture projection of your bones on a film plate. These can be taken while you are lying down or standing up. Doctors may order specific X-rays based on what they want to look at around the hip. X-rays show the bones in detail but do not show the soft tissues, such as muscles, tendons, or ligaments. They represent a shadow of your bony anatomy.

In rare cases, if the hip arthritis is not severe on X-ray, the doctor may order an MRI (magnetic resonance imaging) to see if something else around the hip may be causing pain or dysfunction. MRIs do not use radiation but use magnets to produce a three-dimensional image. An MRI is not as good at showing gross bone anatomy, but it provides additional detail regarding surrounding tissues and helps with a diagnosis of bursitis, tendinitis, or other conditions. However, good X-rays are all that is typically needed to diagnose arthritis.

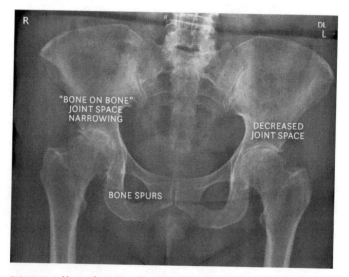

FIGURE 1.4. X-ray depicting "bone on bone" joint space narrowing (*left*) and decreased joint space (*right*) of the hip

Most cases of hip arthritis can be seen on X-rays. Your doctor or surgeon may not need any other tests in order to diagnose you with hip arthritis. Arthritis is diagnosed on X-rays by seeing changes in the bone, including bone spurs or cysts, or less-than-normal space in the hip joint. Cartilage, muscles, tendons, and ligaments cannot be seen on X-rays. If your doctor thinks that there may be another cause of your pain, he or she may order an MRI to look for changes in the cartilage, muscles, ligaments, or tendons.

Your doctor may order blood tests before surgery to evaluate blood counts, blood sugar, kidney function, and ability of the blood to clot. These tests will be discussed in further detail in chapter 3.

Points to Remember

- Simply put, arthritis is wear and tear of our joints over time, specifically causing damage to the normally smooth, slippery cartilage surfaces.

- There are three main types of arthritis: osteoarthritis (OA), inflammatory arthritis such as rheumatoid arthritis (RA), and post-traumatic arthritis. OA is the most common type of arthritis and is a degenerative process, which gets worse slowly over time due to repetitive stress on the joint.

- Pain and stiffness are the main symptoms of hip OA. The pain from hip arthritis is typically located in the groin or buttock.

- X-rays are the main test used to diagnose hip arthritis. In most cases, good X-rays are the only test needed to diagnose hip arthritis.

- Your surgeon should treat you as an individual and not an X-ray. Imaging does not always correlate with symptoms—so even if your arthritis looks severe on X-ray, there is no need for a total hip replacement if you are doing quite well and do not have much pain.

- Initial evaluation by your surgeon will include a discussion of your symptoms, medical conditions, medicines, prior surgeries, and allergies. Quitting smoking prior to surgery can greatly improve your recovery.

- Before even considering hip replacement surgery, nonsurgical strategies to manage the pain and stiffness should be tried. These include weight loss, nonsteroidal anti-inflammatories (NSAIDs), steroid injections, physical therapy, and cane or walker use. How much pain relief you will get from these nonsurgical options is hard to predict. If these nonsurgical options once worked for you but don't anymore, it may be time to have hip replacement surgery.

CHAPTER 2

Is Total Hip Replacement Right for You?

Travis Blood, MD, and Roy K. Aaron, MD

Surgery is rarely the first choice for hip arthritis. There are many nonsurgical ways to minimize pain, from activity modifications and weight loss to nonsteroidal anti-inflammatory drugs (NSAIDs) and finally to more invasive techniques such as joint injections. Once all nonoperative options have been used, it is then reasonable to consider total hip joint replacement, or arthroplasty, as an option.

Once the decision for surgery has been made, your surgeon may recommend other medical evaluations by your primary care doctor. If you see specialists for cardiovascular or respiratory problems, they may also be consulted. Once the proper preoperative exams are completed, you must select a date for surgery. A total hip replacement is an elective procedure, so the timing of surgery depends on when it is right for you. A total hip arthroplasty is a great surgery for the right patient, so be sure it is the right operation for you.

Alternatives to Surgery

Hip pain can be more severe than pain in other joints, negatively affecting normal function, and, therefore, patients can be quite motivated to find relief. There are a number of treatment options that are commonly available to alleviate the pain and disability caused by hip arthritis prior to considering surgical intervention. In some cases, your surgeon may believe that your arthritis is too advanced to try these measures, but in many situations these treatments are viable options. None of these options cure the condition. However, the main goal of each is to relieve some of your pain.

It is rare for a surgeon to recommend surgery as the only option on your first encounter. However, there are some situations where the arthritis is so advanced that the surgeon may feel that nonoperative treatment will not reduce your pain. In these conditions, the surgeon may give you two options. The first option would be to undergo a total hip replacement, and the second option would be to live with the discomfort and try anti-inflammatory medications with the hope of reducing the pain.

Lifestyle Changes

The goal of lifestyle changes is to modify your activities in order to protect your hip and reduce your pain. Limiting activities such as frequently going up and down stairs, running, jumping, and other activities that put high stress across your hip joint can help. Incorporating activities like walking, swimming, and biking into a daily exercise routine puts less stress on your hips compared to higher-impact exercise.

Staying active and doing low-impact exercises keeps your muscles loose and may even decrease your pain. Activities such as running and jumping should be avoided. However, walking, biking, and swimming are great ways to remain active while keeping your flexibility. Additionally, the number-one predictor of your range of motion following surgery is your preoperative range of motion. If you have good preoperative range of motion, you should expect a promising outcome.

Exercise

Low-impact exercise helps maintain your hip range of motion and flexibility and also aids in maintaining the muscle mass of your legs, which is essential if a hip replacement is necessary. Some studies suggest that exercise may even help slow the rate of progression of arthritis. Low-impact exercises like walking, aquatic exercises, and biking have many health benefits, including improving circulation, relieving pain, and increasing muscle tone. In advanced arthritis, exercise can sometimes increase pain. If this occurs, discuss it with your doctor.

Physical Therapy

Specific exercises can help increase your range of motion and flexibility. The goal of physical therapy is to strengthen the supporting muscles of the hip and leg to help reduce pain, stiffness, and swelling. Preoperative physical therapy, or "prehab," may also improve available range of motion and strength in the affected leg, which may subsequently improve postoperative outcomes or expedite recovery if you do have surgery. A physical therapist can tailor a program to your individual needs. Once you are comfortable with your program, you can do the exercises on your own at home.

Weight Loss

Losing weight can make a big difference for many people. Losing weight can result in significant pain relief and a substantial increase in function. Your body mass index (BMI) is a calculation of your weight divided by the square of your height (kg/m²). If your

BMI is greater than 40, your surgeon may recommend a weight loss program for you before proceeding with any surgery. This is because complication rates are significantly increased for people who have a BMI at or above 40. The specific physical distribution of your weight (belly, thighs, buttock) may also influence your surgeon's decision to postpone surgery until after weight loss due to safety concerns at the time of surgery.

Losing weight decreases the forces on your hip, which may alleviate some of your pain. Many people are under the impression that they can't lose weight because their pain makes them unable to exercise, but the reality is that a well-balanced and -monitored diet is the most important step for achieving weight loss. Many dietitians believe that weight loss is 80 to 90 percent diet and 10 to 20 percent exercise.

Assistive Devices

Using an assistive device, such as a cane, may provide substantial symptom relief. A cane can help reduce the amount of pressure across the hip when you walk and should be used in the hand opposite the affected hip. A cane can also help with stability if you are having problems with balance. Using a long-handled grabber to pick things up off the ground may help reduce some pain from bending.

Medications

Medications for arthritis are classified as reducing pain and inflammation (symptom-modifying) or affecting the course of the disease (disease-modifying). For osteoarthritis (OA), disease-modifying medications are not yet available. There are several medications that can be used to help treat the pain of arthritis. Non-narcotic pain relievers and anti-inflammatory medications are usually tried first and are often effective in reducing arthritic pain. Simple pain relievers such as acetaminophen (Tylenol) are available without prescription and can aid in pain control.

NSAIDs are a class of medications that are also available both over the counter and by prescription and help reduce pain and inflammation. They include aspirin, ibuprofen (Motrin or Advil), and naproxen (Aleve). It is important to take these medications with food or as "enteric coated" tablets, as NSAIDs can upset the stomach and lead to serious complications such as bleeding ulcers if not monitored. If you take blood thinners or have a history of gastrointestinal bleeding, you should consult your primary care physician before taking these medications. Your doctor may recommend an additional medication to protect the lining of your stomach.

Cyclooxygenase-2 (COX-2) inhibitors are medications similar to NSAIDs but may have fewer gastrointestinal side effects. Celecoxib (Celebrex) and meloxicam (Mobic, a partial COX-2 inhibitor) are

NSAIDs (nonsteroidal anti-inflammatory drugs) are very powerful medications and are often overlooked as a cause of stomach discomfort. It is very important to take these medications with food to prevent stomach distress. If you develop symptoms, consult your doctor and stop taking these medications, because in extreme cases, the irritation of the stomach can progress to bleeding from the stomach wall. **If bleeding does occur, please contact your local emergency department immediately.**

commonly prescribed to reduce pain and inflammation. You should not take NSAIDs and COX-2 inhibitors at the same time, because they work in similar ways and you could overdose. It is fine, however, to take acetaminophen with NSAIDs and COX-2 inhibitors. Consult with your primary physician prior to taking COX-2 inhibitors if you have had a heart attack, stroke, angina, blood clot, or hypertension.

Specific Disease Medications

For certain types of arthritis, like rheumatoid and psoriatic arthritis, specific medications have been designed to slow the progression of the disease. Disease-modifying antirheumatic drugs (DMARDs), such as methotrexate, sulfasalazine, and hydroxychloroquine, are commonly used to slow the progression of rheumatoid arthritis. Other DMARDs, such as etaner-cept (Enbrel) and adalimumab (Humira), work by reducing the body's immune response and are also commonly prescribed for these conditions. Your primary care physician or a rheumatologist usually prescribes these special medications.

Narcotics

Narcotics (opioids) are seldom prescribed for long-term pain relief from arthritis. Narcotic medications, although effective for pain relief, have many potential side effects, including nausea, vomiting, slowed breathing, constipation, and sleep disturbance. In addition to these side effects, narcotic medications can be extremely addictive; therefore, they should be used with caution. Common narcotic medications are oxycodone-acetaminophen (Percocet), hydrocodone-acetaminophen (Vicodin), oxycodone, and hydrocodone. Tramadol (Ultram) is a synthetic, non-opioid-derived analgesic. Some physicians will have you sign an agreement, or "pain contract," outlining how long you will take these medications, because of their addictive properties. Many states now require a mandatory screening process prior to providing patients with narcotics or restrict how many pills can be prescribed by a physician. In most cases, it is best to limit these medications to short-term use, only for a specific period of time after surgery. The nation-wide opioid crisis has placed increased scrutiny on

Narcotic medications have been highly scrutinized over the last several years. Many physicians are under a lot of pressure to decrease the quantity and duration of opioid medication they prescribe. Many surgeons use a combination of pain treatment methods to limit the amount of narcotics you take and decrease the chances of you becoming addicted to the medication. It is believed that addiction to opioids may begin as early as three days after starting the medication, and using opioids for more than a week is a significant risk factor for addiction.

physicians and surgeons prescribing these narcotics and has renewed interest among prescribers and health organizations in minimizing the dosage and duration of narcotic treatment, even after surgical procedures. Becoming addicted to opioids can cause serious, life-threatening harm. However, they are safe to take during a specific, prescribed period of time after surgery.

Glucosamine and Chondroitin Sulfate

Glucosamine and chondroitin sulfate are naturally occurring compounds within the cartilage of the hip, and these substances are available over the counter without a prescription. Although some people report symptomatic relief after taking them, no clear evidence supports the use of these two dietary supplements for reversal or slowing of hip arthritis. These medications have few side effects, so you may take them with little risk if you choose, but they can be expensive.

Injections

Corticosteroids (also known as cortisone)

Steroids are powerful anti-inflammatory medications that can be injected directly into the painful joint. In some instances, corticosteroids are given orally, but local injection is thought to have a more beneficial effect when treating arthritic pain. Steroid injections reduce pain and inflammation in the joint but do not slow the progression of disease, nor is their beneficial effect permanent. The duration of pain relief between injections is variable, and in many cases you will require multiple injections per year in order to control the pain. Injections in the hip joint are usually done with X-ray or ultrasound guidance, as the actual joint space is deep inside your pelvis. Some surgeons will refer you to a radiologist, while others perform the procedure themselves. If you have diabetes, you may see a rise in your glucose levels for a few days following a steroid injection, and you should use your medications to control this following your primary care provider's advice. Viscosupplements, or "gel injections," are not currently approved by the Food and Drug Administration (FDA) for the hip, because they are for knees; therefore, viscosupplements are not commonly used in managing hip arthritis.

Steroid injections are often referred to as cortisone injections. Many of the steroids used today are derivatives of cortisone but are not truly cortisone. After receiving your hip injections, you may get a local flare reaction. This may result in the area of the injection becoming warm, red, and swollen. The best treatment is to place ice on the hip and monitor it for a few days. Many patients are nervous about infection. However, infection after hip injections are rare. So long as you see improvement in the redness and swelling over the next few days, this is not an infection.

Deciding on Surgery

Hip replacement surgery generally has more predictably good and quicker outcomes than total knee replacement, but keep in mind that the procedure is entirely elective. No doctor should ever tell you that you *must* have your hip replaced. In most cases, the doctor will recommend or advise you that you will likely benefit from a hip replacement when you are ready. Deciding on when to have your hip replaced depends on many factors and varies from person to person. The main purpose of surgery is to eliminate or reduce pain, preserve movement, add stability, and increase function. Many choose to have the surgery when they have significant problems with daily activities such as walking, climbing stairs, putting on their shoes and socks, getting off the toilet, or getting in and out of a bed or car.

Not all sources of hip pain are related to arthritis. Make sure that you discuss your symptoms clearly with your surgeon and that your surgeon considers all possibilities for your given symptoms. Hip pain can originate from nerve irritation in your back, muscle strains, and even abdominal conditions like hernias. The surgeon needs to rule out other sources of pain prior to your making the decision for a total hip replacement.

> **No doctor should ever tell you that you need to have your hip replaced.** In most cases, the doctor will recommend or advise you that you will likely benefit from a hip replacement when you are ready.

Time for a Hip Replacement?

One of the main reasons to consider a hip replacement is to reduce pain that limits everyday activities despite the aid of medications and other nonsurgical strategies. If your hip pain is constant and you are unable to sleep at night, then this may also be a good time to consider a replacement. Some patients feel that they are ready for joint replacement when they can no longer tolerate the pain, while others believe they are ready when they cannot take their nightly walk. In each case, it has to be the right time for you.

Remember **that the best time for surgery is when YOU as the patient are ready**. You need to make sure that you have the proper support from your family and friends before undergoing this operation, as it is a big undertaking and you will need both physical and psychological support. The surgery is the easy part of a hip replacement. Your recovery and time spent in physical therapy are the keys for a great outcome. Therefore, if you can dedicate your time and energy to both of these, your surgery will likely be a success.

After you have tried nonsurgical treatment and feel that you can no longer tolerate the pain, you should consider the possibility of a hip replacement. Discuss the timing of your surgery with your surgeon and any of your close family members and friends who will be helping you through your recovery. The surgery itself takes only a few hours, but the recovery process and rehabilitation take several months and require time and energy for you to get the best possible result. Other things that need to be taken into consideration prior to surgery are time away from work, upcoming holidays, family events, and so on. Sitting down with family members and friends prior to surgery and discussing what works best for all is advisable. Things to consider prior to scheduling a joint replacement surgery are:

- planning time out of work
- travel plans
- family events
- sick leave
- insurance status

Remember that a hip replacement is an elective procedure, and you do not need to rush into the surgery. Having everything in order and well planned will make your recovery process smoother and the process more manageable, and it will probably lead to a better outcome for you.

Although total hip replacement is a common surgery, it comes with some risk, as do all surgical

Once you have decided on having a total hip replacement, it is important to make the correct decision on the right surgeon for you. The comfort and trust you share with your operating surgeon are very important to having a successful outcome. If you do not feel comfortable with a surgeon, it is okay to obtain a second opinion. Any surgeon who is offended by a patient getting a second opinion is not the right surgeon for you. Having confidence in your surgeon will make you feel at ease with the procedure and the rehabilitation process, which is crucial for a great outcome.

procedures. Complications such as deep vein thrombosis (DVT) or blood clots are rare but do happen. Nerve injury is also rare but possible, as is a skin or deep joint infection. It is common that patients and their therapists will notice that the leg with the hip replacement is somewhat longer after the surgery. Dislocation, where the ball of the femur "pops out" of the hip socket, can also occur, especially in the first two months after the operation. The leg with the hip replacement may remain weak after surgery. Changes in the way you walk or favor your leg after surgery may also cause or accelerate problems with your other leg. Although the results of total hip replacement, including pain relief, are often more predictable compared to total knee replacement, the procedure should only be considered when you are willing to take the risk. When the pain is no longer tolerable, surgery is often very successful in providing relief. However, in some rare instances, complications may occur.

Medical Clearance

Prior to surgery, your doctor may request that you see your primary care doctor for preoperative evaluation and "clearance." Because your primary care doctor knows your medical history best, it is advisable to schedule an appointment to be evaluated prior to surgery. At this visit, be sure to tell your primary care physician that you are there for a preoperative clearance appointment. This will allow your doctor to focus on key aspects of your health to prepare you for surgery. In some cases, your primary care doctor may recommend obtaining further testing or further consultation with another specialist prior to surgery. The preoperative clearance is very important, because although total joint replacement is commonly successful, there are rare complications associated with doing the procedure. The purpose of the preoperative checkup is to reduce the risk of these complications as much as possible. In some cases, your surgeon may recommend that you see a cardiologist (heart specialist), nephrologist (kidney specialist), or another specialist. Obtaining medical clearance and optimizing your medications before surgery can lead to a better chance of success without complications.

A total hip replacement is a common procedure across the world. However, as with any surgery, there can still be significant risks. Risks of surgery range from urinary tract infection to blood clots in the lungs and even death. Therefore, it is essential to obtain proper preoperative management prior to surgery. Your surgeon may ask you to obtain medical clearance before surgery to make sure you are as safe as possible. Without proper clearance from medical doctors, your surgeon may refuse to perform the surgery.

Points to Remember

- Total hip replacement should rarely be your first option when considering relief of your hip pain. Prior to visiting a surgeon, try weight loss, exercise, and anti-inflammatory medications to see if these minimally invasive options can reduce the pain.

- Losing weight decreases the forces on your hip, which may alleviate some of your pain. Many people believe that they can't lose weight because their pain keeps them from exercising, but a well-balanced and -monitored diet is the most important step for achieving weight loss.

- Medications for arthritis are classified as slowing or even reversing the course of the disease. Non-narcotic pain relievers and anti-inflammatory medications are usually the first line of treatment. Simple over-the-counter pain relievers can aid in pain control. Narcotic medications should be avoided prior to surgery as they increase postoperative pain and make pain control difficult after surgery while also having high addictive potential.

- Once all nonoperative management has been tried with limited success, then a total hip replacement should be considered. One of the main reasons to consider a hip replacement is to reduce pain that interferes with and limits everyday activities despite the aid of medications and other nonsurgical strategies. If the hip pain is constant and you are unable to sleep at night, then this may be a good time to consider a replacement.

- A total hip replacement is an elective procedure, and proper planning for your surgery and rehabilitation is essential. Discuss the timing of your surgery with your surgeon and any of your close family members and friends who will be helping you through your recovery. The surgery itself only takes a few hours, but the recovery process and rehabilitation take several months and require time and energy for you to get the best possible result.

- Though total hip replacement is a common surgery, it comes with some risks.

- Your surgeon may recommend that you visit your primary care doctor or a specialist for preoperative clearance prior to surgery. This is important to make your surgery as safe as possible.

CHAPTER 3

Preparing for Total Hip Replacement

Matthew E. Deren, MD, and Lee E. Rubin, MD

Preparing for a total hip arthroplasty involves actions by both the patient and potential caregivers, including everything from arranging furniture in the living space to not eating anything on the morning of surgery. Most patients can now safely return home from the hospital rather than being discharged to a skilled nursing facility for rehabilitation. Therefore, preparing meals in advance and arranging help with everyday tasks is important. Speaking with your primary medical physician prior to surgery is important for understanding which medications you should take before surgery. The night before surgery often involves washing the area of your body that will be operated on with a special soap to help prevent infections. You should follow the preoperative directions given to you by your hospital; however, a general rule is that you should have nothing to eat or drink after midnight prior to the day of your surgery.

On the morning of your surgery, you should be brought to the hospital by someone. You should avoid bringing any valuables to the hospital with you. There, you will meet a team of professionals including nurses, anesthesiologists, surgical technologists, physician assistants, and surgeons, who all work together for your surgery. You will be given antibiotics through an intravenous line (IV) to decrease the risk of infection. In the operating room, sterile instruments will be used for your surgery.

Home Preparation

At home, a little preparation can be very helpful for the healing period. Any loose carpets or throw rugs that might cause you to trip should be moved or secured. All chairs, couches, and coffee tables should be arranged to leave space for walking easily between them. Any children's toys should be put away, and small objects on the ground should be removed if possible. Each room that you will spend time in should have a telephone or a charger for your portable or cellular phone, so that you can easily reach friends or family. Do not clean your floors with any detergent that leaves a slippery residue that might cause you to fall. If there are any areas of your house that you are concerned about while recovering from surgery, you can always take a photograph with your cellular phone to show to the physical therapist in the hospital. Then, you both can work on strategies to deal with these challenges when you arrive home after the surgery.

In the kitchen, preparing a few meals in advance and freezing them for later use is a great way to eat well with minimal effort during your recovery phase.

Your house should be prepared for your return home after surgery before you leave for the hospital. This means cleaning up wide-open spaces for you to walk through while you recover. Many people will prepare and freeze meals in advance to make cooking easier during recovery. Also, note how many stairs you will need to climb at home to get into your house and to the room in which you will be sleeping. The physical therapists at the hospital will need this information to help you develop a plan for safely returning home from the hospital.

Determine a place where you will keep all your medications after surgery so that you remember to take them every morning. Some people find it helpful to place the medications or a note near the coffee maker. Buying milk and other drinks in small containers makes it easier to get these out of the refrigerator while holding onto a cane, walker, or crutch with the other hand. Lastly, make sure that pots, pans, and containers that you will use frequently are in cabinets that are easy to reach, rather than in the top or bottom cabinets that would require a step stool or deep bending. Having a large water bottle is a good idea as well, to remind yourself to stay hydrated during your recovery.

Friends and family are essential in successful recovery after a total hip replacement. Creating a list on paper with all important phone numbers, or better yet, saving all these to your phone, is a great idea in case the need for help arises. Often, friends will want to visit in the time after surgery. These visits are best scheduled during the daytime, as you will need to use your evenings to rest and recover from the day's therapy. Your body needs time to heal by resting, and nighttime is the best time for this. Do place night-lights in the hallway and bathroom to illuminate the pathway to the toilet, and keep the floor clear. This is critical to help reduce the risk of falls, which often occur at home while walking to the bathroom at night.

As your recovery can be tough on you, it can also be very difficult for your partner, spouse, or friend. These individuals are your best help, and they are not accustomed to seeing you recovering, so do express your

Saving the phone numbers of your friends and family in your phone (or on a note card) is a good way to ensure that you have these numbers in case the need for help arises. Visits from family members are best during the day, especially during meal times, so that they do not interfere with your physical therapy. Getting good sleep at night helps you recover and work better with therapy the following day. Hospitals can be very difficult to sleep in, so bringing a sleep mask and ear plugs can be very helpful to block out light and noise while you're trying to sleep.

thanks and appreciation for their help. You will need help with household tasks in the first couple of weeks following surgery. Ask friends and family to help with picking up the mail and newspaper daily, assisting with pets, getting groceries, bringing trash and recycling to the curb, and helping with laundry. Without a doubt, receiving help with these chores can make your recovery much less stressful.

Everyone who undergoes hip replacement will receive physical therapy prior to going home after surgery. With current physical therapy and pain control regimens, many people can be discharged directly to their home following surgery, sometimes without even staying overnight in the hospital. Not going to a rehabilitation center or nursing facility following surgery may decrease the risk of developing some infections. Many surgeons prefer that their patients are discharged home following surgery but do realize that preparation and a strong support structure are important to managing at home safely. Some people do benefit from going to a facility after surgery, and this should be something that you consider before having your surgery.

Self-Preparation

Beginning one week prior to surgery, you should begin eating high-fiber foods to avoid constipation before and after surgery and stay as regular as possible with your bowel movements. At your preadmission testing, if this is performed, your doctor will review your list of medications and explain which medications to stop and which to continue. Some medications are very important to your health and need to be taken even on the day of surgery with a sip of water, while others should not. In general, non-prescription vitamins and mineral supplements can be stopped a week prior to the surgery. This is a very good question to ask at your final office visit with both your surgeon and your primary care provider.

Be sure to ask your doctors, both primary care and orthopedic, which medications you should continue, stop, or take a smaller dose of prior to surgery. Some medications are very important to keep your heart healthy during surgery, while others can cause increased bleeding. It is best to have clear instructions on all of these medications at your preoperative appointment and take clear notes on which to continue and when to stop others. On the morning of surgery, you may take your pills with a small sip of water but should not eat or drink anything else.

If you develop a cut, scrape, sore, small infection, pimples, or rash near your operative site, let your surgeon know in advance. Sometimes these can interfere with the surgical incision or may cause your surgery to be delayed for your own safety to prevent wound problems or infection. It is best to be honest and forthright with your surgeon ahead of time if you do notice any of these. Many will cancel a surgery if they notice such a problem that may negatively impact your recovery. Sometimes this will even happen in the preoperative holding area! It's better to give them this information in advance with a call to the office.

If you normally shave the area of your hip where your replacement will be performed, it is best not to do that in the week prior to surgery. Shaving with a razor causes small cuts to the skin, which may allow bacteria in. Under normal circumstances your immune system handles this without any problems, but it can cause a slightly increased risk of skin or deep joint infection when undergoing a joint replacement, so to be safe, leave the area unshaven. Your nurses, doctors, or the operating room assistants will trim the hair close to the skin on the day of surgery with a sterile clipper that will not damage your skin.

Lastly, try to stay relaxed. Total hip replacements are big surgeries, but they are safe and help patients tremendously. Serious complications (such as joint infection) occur in fewer than 2 percent of patients.

The Night before Surgery

The night before surgery, you should try to get a good night's sleep if possible. Take the medications that were reviewed with your primary doctor and at your pre-admission testing visit the night and morning before surgery. You should eat a normal dinner and continue to drink water until bedtime, but do not have anything to eat or drink after midnight. This is to allow the food and drink in your stomach to be digested and travel further into your intestines so that you cannot vomit before, during, or after surgery. You can take your morning pills with a small sip of water.

The evening before and the morning of surgery, you will likely be asked to shower and then rinse your torso and extremities for five minutes with a chlorhexidine 4% soap, such as Hibiclens. Some hospitals use chlorhexidine wipes, which also clean the skin of bacteria. This helps to reduce the number of bacteria living on your skin and therefore reduce the risk of surgical site infection. Sleeping with clean sheets in addition to wearing clean underwear and pajamas are helpful. Lastly, it is best to avoid having pets sleep in your bed for the few days leading up to surgery after you put fresh sheets on the bed.

You can pack a bag of things to bring with you to the hospital. At the very least, consider bringing your

Most hospitals have a protocol for cleaning the skin over your surgical site, beginning prior to your arrival at the hospital on the day of surgery. This helps to reduce the number of bacteria on your skin prior to surgery. This may include chlorhexidine soap. Rarely, people experience irritation of their skin from this soap. If this is the case for you, make sure that you discuss this with your surgeon at your preoperative appointment. There may be another soap you can use that will not cause irritation of your skin. Nearly all people have no trouble with the chlorhexidine soap.

insurance card and identification, as well as a method for making any copayments if required. It is best not to bring large amounts of cash or expensive jewelry with you. You should also bring a copy of your health care directive or power of attorney for medical decision-making for the hospital records. If you own and use a continuous positive airway pressure (CPAP) device for sleep apnea, you should bring this to use at night while you sleep in the hospital.

Many people find it helpful to bring a comfortable pair of shoes with nonskid soles to wear during physical therapy sessions. You can also bring underwear, socks, and some loose-fitting pants (like sweatpants) to wear that still allow access to the bandage. Having your glasses, hearing aids, and dentures will support your recovery by letting you return to normal as quickly as possible. Many people find that their lips are chapped following surgery, so having lip balm or sucking hard candy might make you more comfortable. You can also bring some magazines or books to read in your free time as you recover after surgery.

As mentioned above, it is best not to bring large amounts of cash to the hospital. If you would like to use a Kindle, iPad, tablet, or laptop computer following surgery, a family member or friend can bring these to you after surgery, but it is best not to bring them to the operating room at the time of your surgery. Almost all of the medications that you normally take at home are available from the hospital pharmacy; therefore, you do not need to bring your own medications unless you take a very unusual drug. Ask your surgeon about this before surgery. Likewise, canes, walkers, and crutches will be provided by your physical therapists during your stay, so usually you do not need to bring these devices to the hospital at the time of your surgery. You should not place any marks or initials anywhere on your extremities, as these will have to be removed per hospital protocol.

The last thing you need on the day of surgery is a ride! You will not be allowed to drive yourself home from the hospital; therefore, you should have someone drop you off on the day of surgery and plan to have someone pick you up on the day you are leaving. If your surgery is planned as a "same-day" or "outpatient" procedure, this person will need to be available in the afternoon to take you home from the hospital.

You should only bring the essentials that you need to the operating room at the time of your surgery, including a comfortable pair of shoes to wear during physical therapy as well as an identification card and your health insurance card. Avoid bringing expensive jewelry, laptops, or tablets to the operating room. A friend or family member can bring these to your room in the hospital after your surgery is complete. Keep in mind that you will have to remove all jewelry during surgery and change into a hospital gown. Glasses, dentures, and hearing aids are important to bring with you and will be removed but safely stored during surgery. These items allow you to see, chew, and hear before and after surgery, so be sure to bring them!

Points to Remember

- Preparing your home for your return after surgery is essential for a safe recovery. This includes preparing and freezing meals, installing night-lights, clearing clutter, and asking for help with basic activities like getting the mail and doing laundry.

- Be sure to ask your doctor which medications should be continued, stopped, or taken at a smaller dose around the time of surgery.

- Follow all directions regarding care of the site of your surgery, including washing the area with a special soap and not shaving it in the week leading up to your surgery.

- Be sure to have a ride, both to and from the hospital!

- Leave expensive jewelry, electronics, and cash at home. Do bring your glasses, dentures, and hearing aids, as well as a comfortable pair of shoes, to help in your recovery.

- Remember to not eat or drink anything after midnight the night before your surgery. On the morning of surgery, take the medications you were instructed to continue with a sip of water and nothing more.

CHAPTER 4

Surgery and Hospital Stay

Scott Ritterman, MD, and John Froehlich, MD, MBA

Arriving at the Hospital

On the day of surgery, your first stop will be the hospital registration desk. After checking in, you will proceed to the preoperative area, or holding unit, of the operating room. There, your loved ones will often be able to sit with you until you leave for the operating room itself, at which point they will go to the waiting room.

You should plan to arrive at the hospital roughly two hours prior to your scheduled procedure, according to your surgeon's directions. Usually, you should not eat or drink anything starting at midnight the night before your surgery. If your surgery is later in the day, clear liquids may be allowed until two hours prior to surgery. When you arrive and register, you will be given a name bracelet. Then you will be taken into a changing area, where you can change into a hospital gown. All of your clothing and personal effects will be labeled and put aside until after your procedure. Please remember to leave any valuables, especially jewelry, at home during your hospital stay. Remove all rings, earrings, bracelets, and necklaces before coming to the hospital. If you wear glasses and have a cheaper pair, bring those. If you wear contact lenses, do not wear them on the day of surgery. However, you should bring them with you, along with an extra pair.

After changing, you will move into the preoperative holding area. Here you will get ready for your procedure and meet the members of your surgical team. A nurse will check you in and ask some questions. You will be asked your name, date of birth, what procedure you are having, and on what side it is being performed. While it will seem repetitive, please understand that this repetition is essential to making sure the correct procedure is being performed and avoiding mistakes.

You should plan to arrive at the hospital roughly two hours prior to your scheduled procedure. Your surgeon's office will direct you when and where to show up on the day of surgery. Do not eat or drink anything starting at midnight the night before your surgery. If your surgery is later in the day, clear liquids may be allowed until two hours prior to surgery.

It is helpful to bring a current list of all the medications you regularly take. Most medications are available in the hospital pharmacy, but your doctor may advise you to bring less common medications with you for your hospital stay.

When you come to the hospital, it is good to have a family member or a friend hold your personal

At the hospital, you will be asked the same questions several times. You will give your name, date of birth, what procedure you are having, and on what side it is being performed. While it will seem repetitive, please understand that everyone has the same goal in mind—getting you through your procedure as safely as possible.

belongings while you are in the operating room. Things to bring with you may include reading material (books or magazines), a cell phone with charger, reading glasses if needed, and a change of loose-fitting clothes that are easy to put on.

The nurse will check your vital signs including your heart rate, blood pressure, breathing rate, and temperature. He or she will also speak to you about your medical history and the surgery you will be having today. The nurse will start an intravenous (IV) line for fluid and medications to be given during surgery.

Team Members

After you are checked in, you will meet several team members while waiting for your procedure. In the operating room, in addition to your surgeon, there will be several people who may assist in the operation. A "circulator" nurse supervises and records events that go on in the operating room. This person is responsible for getting any equipment that is needed during the procedure, opening sterile boxes, and so on. A scrub nurse or scrub technician (tech) is responsible for the sterility and management of the surgical tools and implants. They keep the instruments clean, hand the surgeons the required instruments, and keep everything in the operating room sterile.

Nearly all surgical procedures require an assistant who helps the surgeon perform the operation. Teaching hospitals typically include either resident physicians, who have completed medical school and are training to become surgeons, or fellow physicians, advanced

Surgeons rarely perform operations alone, and the entire team is important to the success of your surgery.

Who will be on your team?

- Surgeon
- Circulator nurse, who supervises and records events and gets equipment
- Scrub technician
- Surgeon's assistant
- Physician's assistant
- Representative from vendor that supplies implant devices

trainees who have completed an orthopedic surgical residency and are training in one particular specialty of their field, such as hip replacement surgery. Physician assistants help physicians in both the operating room as well as the office and may assist in your surgery. Additionally, there are nurses who assist in some hospitals or surgery centers. If you have any questions or concerns about who may be helping in your surgery, please discuss these with your surgeon directly.

Many operating rooms will also have a vendor representative from the implant company in the room. These representatives ensure that the hospital is stocked with appropriate surgical components and instruments. They are well versed in their company's implants and are able to ensure the correct devices are being utilized by the nursing staff.

Anesthesia

Your anesthesia provider, either an anesthesiologist (a medical doctor) or a certified registered nurse anesthetist (CRNA), a nurse who has undergone specialized training in anesthesia, will speak with you before your procedure. Their goal is to get you through the operation safely and comfortably. They will take a medical history as well as an anesthesia history. It is important to discuss with them if you get very nauseated coming out of anesthesia or if any family members have had problems with anesthesia in the past. They will also discuss the risks of anesthesia and answer any questions you may have. It is a good idea to write a few questions down to ask beforehand, as you may not remember them on the spot.

The anesthesia provider will ask you to open your mouth and examine your airway. They will also ask you to remove any false teeth and identify any loose teeth, caps, crowns or problem areas. Damage to the teeth during intubation is very rare but is a risk of undergoing general anesthesia. They will start an intravenous line (IV) in either your hand, forearm, or inner elbow.

The two main types of anesthesia are general anesthesia and spinal anesthesia. General anesthesia means that you will be asleep during the procedure and a tube will be placed into your windpipe so you can breathe during the procedure (you will not be aware of this!). Your breathing will be aided by a machine that delivers anesthetic gas and measures the size and rate of your breaths to ensure you have enough oxygen.

Spinal anesthesia is a form of regional anesthesia whereby medication is introduced into the area around the spinal nerves in your back. This medication blocks nerve signals to and from the lower half of your body during the procedure. You will not be able to move or feel your legs throughout the surgery and for several hours afterward. Spinal anesthesia can be an "awake" surgery, meaning that your level of consciousness is not affected and you may be able to hear members of the team talking and working during your procedure. More commonly, light sedation, or "twilight" anesthesia, is combined with spinal anesthesia to sedate you during the procedure.

There are two types of anesthesia:

1. General anesthesia
2. Spinal anesthesia, for "awake surgery"

If your surgeon uses spinal anesthesia and you do not want to be awake during your procedure, this is something you can discuss with the anesthesia team before surgery. Likewise, if you are uncomfortable with spinal anesthesia altogether, discuss your concerns with your surgeon before the day of surgery.

Finally, some surgeons use a combination of several medications injected directly into the tissues surrounding the hip joint during your procedure. These medications may include a local anesthetic, an anti-inflammatory, and a pain reliever. This can help control pain after the procedure.

Once you are fully checked in and have been seen by both the anesthesiologist and your surgeon, you are ready for the operating room. When the room is set up and ready, you will be rolled in a stretcher or bed down to the operating room for your surgery.

In the Operating Room

After arriving in the operating room (OR), you will meet the operating room circulating nurse as well as the surgical technologist who helps the surgeon with the tools needed for the procedure. Other staff, such as orderlies, anesthesia technicians, or equipment and surgical technology representatives, may be present. Often, there can be 8 to 10 people in the operating room working with you and the surgeon throughout the procedure. Each one of these professionals plays a unique and important role.

You may or may not remember your journey to the operating room due to the sedation that is given through the IV line. Once in the OR, you will be moved over to the operating room table. In virtually all institutions, you will be checked in and identified once again. Once all the prerequisite checks are completed, the anesthesiologist will either induce general anesthesia or position you for spinal anesthesia. Once you are under anesthesia, you will be positioned for the procedure. Regardless of the position you are placed in, careful attention will be made to pad all the bony prominences and pressure points over nerves in your body. If you have a joint or extremity that is stiff or does not have full normal motion, you should mention it to the nurse before the procedure, to make sure it will be positioned comfortably.

You will be given antibiotics through your IV prior to the start of the surgery. This is to prevent bacteria, which live on the surface of everyone's skin, from getting deeper into your tissues and causing an infection. Immediately before the surgery, your skin will be cleansed again with an antiseptic such as chlorhexidine 4% to kill the skin bacteria and reduce the risk of infection.

In some cases, a urinary catheter, or Foley catheter, will be used to allow you to urinate into a container during the procedure. This prevents your bladder from becoming too full and lets the medical team keep track of your body fluid status. This is dependent on the procedure and the surgeon, so you may not have one. If needed, this is typically placed after anesthesia has been administered. In some cases this will be removed at the end of the surgery, before you wake up from anesthesia.

The operating room is often kept relatively cool for the comfort of the operating staff, but it is important for you to stay warm during surgery to allow your body to function normally. Because of this, many hospitals use warming blankets and devices that blow heated air onto you to keep you warm during surgery.

The operating room is a sterile environment. Personnel must wear hospital-issued and -cleaned scrubs, hats, and masks within the operating room to maintain this sterile environment. All of the instruments are specially prepared to maintain sterility. **A good rule is that anything blue within the operating room is likely to be sterile.**

Surgical Approaches

There are a number of different ways to perform a total hip replacement, including different surgical approaches. Some surgeons use X-ray guidance, computer navigation, or robotic assistance, while others rely on their knowledge of anatomy and their surgical expertise alone.

An approach is just as it sounds, the direction and path taken to get to the hip joint to safely perform a hip replacement. Each approach to the hip requires spreading between or splitting different muscles. While some surgeons prefer one approach to another, large studies have demonstrated that the longer-term outcomes of all approaches are similar. Most surgeons use the approach they are trained in and feel most comfortable using.

The posterior approach is a very common and safe approach for total hip replacement but may be associated with an increased risk of postoperative hip dislocation when compared to other approaches. The lateral approach to the hip, or the anterolateral approach, has a very good track record for stability; however, it requires the surgeon to detach and then repair tendons in the strong hip muscles called the abductors, which may result in postoperative weakness, a limp, or muscle problems. Finally, the direct anterior approach has the benefit of low dislocation rates without the need to detach any muscles or tendons, but it can have a higher risk of skin numbness adjacent to

There are many ways for a surgeon to perform a total hip arthroplasty. Some surgeons use X-ray guidance, computer navigation, or robotic assistance, while others rely on their knowledge of anatomy. Common approaches include

- Posterior approach

- Lateral approach

- Anterolateral approach

- Direct anterior approach

- The best approach for you is probably the approach that your surgeon is most comfortable performing for your unique anatomy and condition.

the incision. The best approach for you is probably the approach that your surgeon is most comfortable performing for your unique anatomy and condition. Many factors are considered in the surgeon's choice of approach, and it might be helpful to discuss this with your surgeon before surgery.

The anterior approach to the hip is performed with the patient lying on their back. Both the lateral and posterior approaches require the patient to be lying on their side. Careful attention is paid to padding any portion of the body that may feel pressure during the procedure.

The specifics of each procedure are different, but the basic steps of a total hip replacement are that both the ball (femoral head) and the socket (acetabulum) are resurfaced. Worn-out cartilage is removed, and the bone is prepared for implant placement. Typically, a stem made of titanium is press-fit into the femur. Press-fit components have special coatings that allow bone to integrate into the implant and grow onto the prosthesis. The initial press-fit during surgery holds the implant in the bone. Over the next few months, the bone will actually grow into the coating of the implant. This process has the advantage of creating a long-lasting bond that can remain stable and strong over time. A prosthetic femoral head made either of cobalt-chrome or ceramic is then placed on top of that stem. The socket is often composed of a titanium-backed metal "cup," or shell, and a polyethylene (high-strength plastic) or ceramic liner.

After surgery, the surface you use for walking and bearing weight on is a metal or ceramic ball on a plastic or ceramic liner. As with natural cartilage, there is very little friction between the two surfaces, which allows for smooth motion and the greatest implant duration of service possible, often 10 to 20 years. Your surgeon will work to recreate the mechanics of your hip joint and to normalize your leg lengths as much as possible.

After Surgery

After your procedure is finished, you will be taken to the recovery room. A nurse will stay with you through the first several hours after your procedure. In the recovery room, your vital signs, such as heart rate, breathing rate, blood pressure, and temperature, will be monitored. Your anesthesia provider will still be responsible for your pain control as well as ensuring a smooth awakening from anesthesia. When you are comfortable, family members will often be allowed to visit with you. Once you have woken and are medically stable and your vital signs are normal, you will be sent to your room to begin your recovery and start using your new hip!

Nursing Staff

When you arrive at your room on the hospital floor you will meet several people. One will be your nurse, an RN (registered nurse). They will be your primary caregiver during your stay. They are responsible for administering medications and can help you with any questions you may have. A certified nurse assistant, or CNA, will also assist your nurse in your care. They may be responsible for ensuring that you have a fresh ice pack for your hip and can help you move to the bathroom. They can get any additional blankets or linens you may need during your stay.

Afternoon of Surgery

If you had surgery early in the day, you will likely be asked to get out of bed on the same day. You may be asked to move to a chair near your bed or even stand

and walk. This is safe to do and actually has been shown to improve your early recovery after the operation. If you are hungry and passing gas, you will be able to have some food. Try to start slowly, as nausea is not uncommon after surgery. Medication for nausea is available if needed. Your family and friends can visit with you in your room after surgery. Be mindful of visiting hours, especially if you are sharing a room with another patient.

Sleeping in the Hospital

You may or may not be able to sleep well the night after your procedure. If you often use earplugs or anything else to help you fall asleep, it would be prudent to bring those with you. Please let your medical team know if you take sleeping medications regularly. If you regularly read before bed, bring a book. Closing the door may be helpful if you are situated near the nurses' station or a particularly noisy part of the nursing unit. Any concerns you may have should be discussed with your nurse. Try to get some sleep, and be prepared to be woken up early (around six o'clock) for morning blood draws.

The Next Morning

You will likely be woken early on the morning after surgery for blood draws. These are typically done to check your blood level as well as the electrolyte

Getting out of bed on the first day after surgery is very important. Getting out of bed helps prevent blood clots in the leg and pneumonia. You should make a plan with your nurse and the physical therapy team to get out of bed several times the first day. Setting small goals will help you progress through your recovery both in the hospital and upon discharge.

concentrations in your blood. It is normal to have some blood loss from surgery. Either before or after breakfast, you should be prepared to get out of bed. Getting out of bed on the first day after surgery is very important. Movement is an essential part of your recovery that helps prevent blood clots in the leg and pneumonia. Once you are up and about, a urinary catheter will be taken out if it was placed for the surgery. Make a plan with your nurse and the physical therapy team to get out of bed several times the first day. Try eating your meals from the chair instead of the bed. Have a goal in mind about how far you want to walk, be it to the door of the room or the nurses' station. Setting small goals will help you progress through your recovery both in the hospital and upon discharge. Once you are eating enough food and taking in water and other fluids, the intravenous fluid can be discontinued. Often an IV will be left in place while you are hospitalized, just in case some medication needs to be delivered quickly.

Blood Transfusions

After surgery, blood draws will be used to measure your blood hemoglobin (the compound in blood that carries oxygen) levels and evaluate whether you may need a blood transfusion. Blood transfusions are becoming less common after hip joint replacement. This is due to a variety of factors, including better control of blood loss during surgery (meticulous hemostasis), use of medications such as tranexamic acid that help reduce blood loss when given before or during surgery, and new research about what levels of hemoglobin are safe.

If your surgeon determines that you do need a blood transfusion, perhaps because you have a low starting hemoglobin concentration before surgery (anemia) or your surgery is more complex, you may be given blood through your IV. Your blood type will be checked, and a sample will be taken to ensure that your blood is compatible with the donor blood you will be getting. Your name should be checked several times against the donated blood that has been selected for you to accurately ensure that it is your blood type. Hospital staff are trained to ensure blood compatibility, but you should look, as well.

Previously, patients would donate blood before surgery so they could receive their own blood after surgery. This is no longer common practice, because studies have found that the donation actually lowers your blood count and increases the likelihood of needing a transfusion.

Pain Management

Understandably, most people are concerned about pain after a hip replacement surgery. Everyone experiences pain differently. Everyone will experience some degree of discomfort after surgery, but this is very different for each person. Realistic expectations are important. To have no pain whatsoever is an unrealistic expectation, but you should be comfortable and able to participate in physical therapy. People who are already taking narcotic pain medications often have a more difficult time with pain management and are at greater risk for narcotic side effects.

Most surgeons now utilize a "multimodal" pain management plan, which includes a series of pills, nerve block injections, and injections around the joint during surgery. This combination helps block pain in a number of different ways. This method may start in the preoperative area, continue during the procedure, and also help control your pain after surgery. Surgeons use a combination of narcotic (opioid) and non-narcotic pain medication. Opioid medications are derived from morphine. These medications have excellent pain reduction properties but do have several drawbacks. They are often short-lasting, meaning that you will require multiple doses every several hours, and they can be habit forming. Non-narcotic pain medications can include acetaminophen (Tylenol) given either through an IV or orally. Other classes of non-narcotic pain medication include nonsteroidal anti-inflammatory medication.

Often patients will receive acetaminophen around the clock, meaning every eight hours, without having to ask for it. Additionally, oxycodone (narcotic pain medication) will be available "on demand" every three to four hours. An IV "rescue" pain medication such as morphine or hydromorphone is also available in the first day or two after surgery. For patients around or over the age of 80 years, narcotic doses are significantly reduced. Please tell your nurse or surgeon if you have previously had a problem with narcotic pain medication, either because of substance abuse, allergic reaction, or if you did not like the way they made you feel. Alternative medications are available.

Physical Therapy

Physical therapy typically starts on the same day as surgery. Expect to get out of bed following surgery and make it to a bedside chair or the toilet. Each day after surgery you should walk a little farther. In the hospital, the main goals are safe movement, gait training (learning to walk again with an assistive device such as a walker or crutches), and regaining balance. Call for help whenever you need to get out of your hospital bed after surgery. To reduce the risk of falling, do not attempt to get out of bed on your own.

The physical therapists will help get you ready for discharge. Discuss any obstacles that you may face getting back into your home. Think about how many stairs you need to climb and whether a railing is available. If possible, attempt to start your recovery on a single floor within your home.

After a total hip replacement, some people will benefit from physical therapy to work on gait, balance training, and strengthening and retraining the muscles used when walking. It is a good idea to figure out where you will go for outpatient physical therapy before your operation if necessary. Surgeons usually have recommendations or "rehab protocols" to help coordinate recovery care with physical therapy providers. You can meet with a physical therapist before your surgery. Picking somewhere close to home that is easy to get to is important. In some cases, with the use of advanced surgical techniques, total hip replacement patients may recover so quickly that prolonged outpatient physical therapy is not prescribed by their surgeon.

Falls after surgery can occur for a variety of reasons, including muscle weakness, long-lasting effects of anesthesia, too much pain medication, or delirium (altered mental status), just to name a few. A fall in the hospital can be very serious, which is why you need to ask for help if you are getting out of bed or moving from the chair.

Hip Precautions

One of the most common complications following a hip replacement is dislocation. In a dislocation, the prosthetic head (the ball) comes out of the cup (the socket). This is usually a painful event, and it is quite obvious when it happens. Some surgeons will place patients on "hip precautions" after surgery to decrease the likelihood of a dislocation.

Depending on the approach to the hip joint used during surgery, your surgeon may place you on anterior, lateral, or posterior hip precautions. For example, anterior hip precautions mean that you should avoid extending, externally rotating, and adducting (bringing your operative leg across the midline of your body) your operative leg (the leg that was operated on). This motion might occur when reaching for a towel when coming out of the shower. Posterior hip precautions mean that you should avoid flexing your hip past 90 degrees and rotating it internally. You should avoid situations that involve bending too much at the hip, such as bending to put on socks and shoes or sitting in a deep chair or bucket-type seat. Lateral hip precautions usually mean no active abduction (moving your leg away from the midline of your body) and no crossing the operative leg over the nonoperative one.

Lateral precautions are meant to protect the repair of soft tissues rather than prevent a dislocation. In general, it is good to avoid extremes of motion after a total hip replacement. Try not to pivot on your operative leg when walking, especially in the first few months after a hip replacement. Different surgeons give different recommendations for hip precautions after surgery or use a defined "protocol." Hip precautions will be discussed in more detail in chapter 5.

Urinary Catheter

Some surgeons will prefer that a urinary catheter is placed during surgery, especially for longer or more complex hip procedures such as operations on patients who have had previous hip surgery. While a urinary catheter can help drain your bladder and prevent urinary retention, if left in place too long, it can also increase your risk of getting a urinary tract infection. Catheters are often removed as soon as you are able to move to urinate comfortably.

If you have a pre-existing problem urinating, either retention or incontinence, you should discuss this with the nurse who checks you in. This is especially important for men with a history of an enlarged prostate, a history of prostate cancer, or anyone with a history of a urethral stricture (decreased size of the opening of the urethra, where urine exits the body). Pain medications, constipation, and pain itself can all lead to urinary retention. In the event that you are unable to go to the bathroom on your own, a catheter may need to be inserted. To determine when your catheter can be removed, you may have a void trial. In a void trial, the catheter is removed, and you try to void (urinate) on your own. If you cannot do so for eight hours, your catheter may have to be replaced, and you may need to be seen by a urologist upon discharge. You may also be checked for a urinary tract infection (UTI) with a urine screening test or a urine culture. Symptoms of an infection may include painful or burning sensations with urination, foul-smelling or cloudy urine, or an inability to control your urine as normal. If you have a urinary tract infection, you will be placed on antibiotics until the infection clears up.

Bowel Regimen

Keeping a normal schedule of bowel movements is important in the days following your procedure. For several reasons, constipation is common following a joint replacement procedure. You will not be eating or drinking as much as normal. Narcotic pain medication often leads to constipation, as can the actual pain itself. It is important to stay hydrated during your hospitalization. Additionally, you will be given several bowel medications after surgery and also upon discharge. If you regularly take medication to improve your bowel habits, writing down exactly what you take or bringing your medication to the hospital is a good idea. If you are unable to make a bowel movement for more than a few days or begin to experience abdominal pain after surgery, call your surgeon for discussion and evaluation.

Antibiotics

Most people receive antibiotics before a hip replacement surgery. As mentioned previously, you should
discuss any medication allergies with team members in
the preoperative area. You may or may not receive further doses of antibiotics after surgery. Infections are a
potentially serious complication of joint replacement
surgery and can have significant and long-lasting con-
sequences. Taking antibiotics before and after surgery
has been shown to decrease the risk of infection.

Pulmonary Toilet

Pulmonary toilet refers to taking deep breaths after
surgery and clearing any mucus that may develop.
After general anesthesia and receiving narcotic pain
medication, the body's breathing center in the brain is
slowed. Breathing problems combined with time spent
in bed can lead to postsurgical atelectasis, or collapse
of the small airways deep within the lung. If untreated,
this can develop into a pneumonia, or bacterial infection within the lungs. Though rare, hospital-acquired
pneumonia is a serious problem after joint replacement surgery.

The best way to prevent both atelectasis and pneumonia is by sitting upright and walking after surgery.
Additionally, sitting up straight while in bed and taking
deep breaths can help. A breathing device called an
"incentive spirometer" may be given to you during your

hospital stay. This helps expand your lungs by encouraging you to take and hold deep breaths.

Deep Vein Thrombosis Prophylaxis

Getting a deep vein thrombosis (DVT) is a major risk of joint replacement surgery. This is a clot that forms in the larger veins of the legs or pelvis and can lead to leg swelling and pain. A pulmonary embolism (PE) is when a blood clot travels through the body and becomes lodged in the veins of the lungs, impairing oxygen delivery to the bloodstream and the body. A large PE can be fatal. The best way to decrease your risk of getting a DVT or PE is to walk several times a day and move around throughout the day. This is especially important during the first four to six weeks after surgery. Additionally, almost all surgeons put patients on some kind of medication to thin the blood, making blood less likely to clot within the veins. However, this puts you at a higher risk of bleeding if you cut yourself or fall. Ask your surgeon what they use for DVT prophylaxis after surgery and for how long. Common options include aspirin (pill), enoxaparin (injection), and warfarin or Coumadin (pill). Coumadin requires having regular blood tests. Newer pill options now also exist. Please discuss with your surgeon if you are already on medications that increase your risk for bleeding. These can include clopidogrel (Plavix), aspirin, and nonsteroidal anti-inflammatory drugs (NSAIDs), among others.

Common risks associated with surgery include

- *Dislocation*, which refers to when the prosthetic head (the ball) comes out of the cup (the socket). Some surgeons will place patients on what is referred to as a "hip precaution" after surgery to decrease the likelihood of a postoperative dislocation.

- *Deep vein thrombosis*, a clot that forms in the larger veins of the legs or pelvis and can lead to leg swelling and pain. A pulmonary embolism (PE) is when a blood clot travels and becomes lodged in the veins of the lung, which impairs oxygen delivery to the bloodstream and the body; a large PE can be fatal.

You may wake up from surgery with a stocking on one or both of your legs. These are designed to compress the veins of the lower leg, preventing swelling and enhancing blood flow back to the heart. Sequential compression devices (SCDs) may also be placed on your feet or calves during your hospitalization. The goal of these devices is to squeeze the muscles of your leg or foot, propelling blood out of your legs toward your heart.

As with pain control, most surgeons utilize a multimodal approach when it comes to DVT prophylaxis. Combining the effects of chemical prophylaxis (medicines), mechanical prophylaxis (SCDs), exercises, and walking around after surgery helps to decrease the chances of developing a DVT or PE.

Visiting Hours

Your family and friends will be able to visit you in your hospital room. Discuss with your nurse and physical therapist when visitors should come so that their visits don't coincide with your physical therapy.

Case Managers

Case managers, also known as care coordinators or navigators, work on inpatient hospital units and facilitate your discharge from the hospital. They help to set up at-home services, such as skilled nursing or physical therapy visits, and order devices such as walkers or canes. This is also a good person to discuss any obstacles to discharge that you may encounter. Case managers can also help facilitate your transfer to a nursing facility if that is where you are planning on going upon discharge.

Discharge from the Hospital

Your discharge from the hospital should be planned well in advance of your procedure. You can either be discharged to home or to a nursing facility. Most people are now discharged directly to home, but a nursing facility may be more appropriate, depending on your medical situation and social support system. If you are planning on going home after your procedure, you should discuss the specific difficulties in getting into and out of your home with your physical therapist. For example, if you live in a second-floor apartment, you will need to work on going up stairs with the in-house physical therapist before being cleared to go home.

Going home is a big responsibility after joint replacement surgery but is very doable. Planning ahead helps. Who is going to help you in the morning? In the evening? Who is going to help you get to the bathroom throughout the day? Who is going to help you shower? These are all questions to think about before your procedure. The level of support you need may not be as high as you expect, but it's best to be prepared.

Points to Remember

- You should plan to arrive at the hospital roughly two hours prior to your scheduled procedure. Do not eat or drink anything starting at midnight the night before your surgery. If your surgery is later in the day, clear liquids may be allowed until two hours prior to surgery.

- Surgeons rarely perform operations alone, and an entire team is necessary for the success of your surgery. Often, there can be 8 to 10 people in the operating room working with you and the surgeon during the procedure. Each one of these professionals plays a unique and important role.

● Your anesthesia provider will speak with you before your procedure. Their goal is to get you through the operation safely and comfortably. It is a good idea to write a few questions down to ask beforehand, as you may not remember them on the spot.

● The operating room is a sterile environment. Personnel must wear hospital-issued and -cleaned shirts, pants, hats, and masks within the operating room to maintain this sterile environment. All of the instruments are specially prepared to maintain sterility.

● There are many ways of performing a total hip replacement. The best approach for you is probably the approach that your surgeon is most comfortable performing for your unique anatomy and condition.

● To have no pain whatsoever is an unrealistic expectation. A more reasonable expectation is for pain control to ensure that you are comfortable and able to participate in physical therapy.

● Going home is a big responsibility after joint replacement surgery but is very doable. Planning ahead and having help are important.

CHAPTER 5

After Surgery

Eric Cohen, MD, and Derek R. Jenkins, MD

Congratulations on your new total hip replacement! This chapter covers postoperative care after you leave the hospital, whether you are going home or to a rehabilitation unit. This section will cover pain management, diet, mood, sleep, gastrointestinal issues, urinary retention, fever, leg swelling, management of a drain, how to take care of your incision, when to resume home medication, and when to resume daily activities, as well as rehabilitation protocols.

Hip Precautions

There are many different surgical approaches for total hip replacement, and each one has been shown to have very good results. Your surgeon may advise you to follow hip precautions as outlined below to prevent hip dislocation. Usually, hip precautions are no longer necessary six weeks after surgery, though general principles are helpful to consider for the lifetime of your hip replacement.

If you had a **posterior** surgical approach hip replacement, you should maintain posterior hip precautions:

- Do not flex your hip past 90 degrees.

- Do not cross your legs past the midline.

- Do not twist your hip or legs inward.

- Keep your feet, toes, and knees facing forward at all times.

If you had a **lateral** surgical approach hip replacement, then you should maintain lateral hip precautions:

- Do not flex your hip past 90 degrees.

- Do not cross your legs past the midline.

- Do not twist your hip or legs inward.

- Keep your feet, toes, and knees facing forward at all times.

- Do not actively abduct your leg (move your leg away from the midline of your body) or undergo

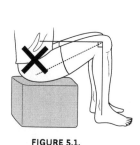

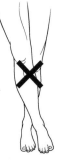

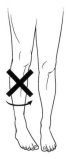

FIGURE 5.1.
Posterior hip precautions:
Don't bend your hip more than 90 degrees

FIGURE 5.2.
Posterior hip precautions:
Don't cross your operative leg past the midline

FIGURE 5.3.
Posterior hip precautions:
Don't turn the leg that was operated on inward.

abduction strengthening exercises for one to three months after surgery, as your surgeon recommends.

If you had an **anterior** surgical approach hip replacement, then you should maintain anterior hip precautions:

- Do not overextend your hip (lean excessively backward).

- Do not cross your legs past the midline.

- Do not "plant and pivot" your operative leg, meaning don't twist or rotate your operative leg outward (especially when leaning backward with your operative side foot planted on the ground).

- Avoid straight leg raise exercises for the first six weeks after surgery.

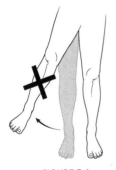 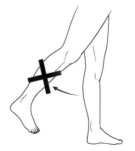 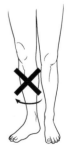

FIGURE 5.4.
Lateral hip precautions:
No active hip abduction
(moving your leg away from
the midline of your body)

FIGURE 5.5.
**Anterior hip
precautions:**
No hip extension

FIGURE 5.6.
**Anterior hip
precautions:**
No external
rotation of the hip

Pain Management

Your orthopedic surgeon will prescribe you a multi-modal pain regimen prior to leaving the hospital; this often includes a combination of acetaminophen (Tylenol), nonsteroidal anti-inflammatory drugs (NSAIDs), and opioid pain medication. Please let your doctor know of any allergies to any such medications prior to leaving the hospital. Follow the prescription label for how much to take of each particular medication, frequency, and side effects. The most powerful pain management medication that you will be prescribed is in the opioid family of medicines and typically includes acetaminophen-oxycodone (Percocet), acetaminophen-hydrocodone (Vicodin), and oxycodone. These are effective for moderate to severe pain and are generally short-acting in nature. These medications can be taken initially to control your pain but then should be taken less frequently over the next two weeks. Opioids work by mimicking your body's natural pain relievers, such as endorphins. The opioids block the pain receptors to your brain and nerves, providing relief, but can also affect your gastrointestinal tract by causing constipation. This is why it is important to take laxatives and stool softeners while taking opioid pain medicine to maintain regular bowel movements. Other side effects are drowsiness, confusion, and itching. You should not drive or operate any heavy machinery while taking narcotic pain medicine.

Opioid medications are important in the immediate postoperative period for pain control but should be taken less frequently over the first two weeks. Every patient's pain perception and pain medication needs are different; however, the goal is to wean off the medication in the early postoperative period. Once you no longer need prescription medications, you need to properly dispose of these medications. Please visit the DEA Diversion Control Divisions website (www.deadiversion.usdoj.gov) for information on National Prescription Drug Take-Back Day events and DEA-authorized collectors, or you may call the DEA Office of Diversion Control's Registration Call Center at 1-800-882-9539 to find an authorized collector in your area.

Another prescription that may be prescribed is an NSAID such as ibuprofen, naproxen, meloxicam, or aspirin. NSAIDs work by preventing prostaglandin production. Prostaglandins are molecules that cause inflammation and pain. There are two important enzymes required to create prostaglandins, COX-1 and COX-2. These enzymes are inhibited by nonsteroidal anti-inflammatory medications, which prevent the production of prostaglandins, decreasing inflammation and pain at the surgery site. There are usually less-severe side effects with anti-inflammatory medications compared to opioid medications; however, there are still important side effects, including gastrointestinal irritation or bleeding. A special class of nonsteroidal anti-inflammatory medications, such as celecoxib (Celebrex), specifically for COX-2 inhibitors, has fewer gastrointestinal side effects.

Acetaminophen (Tylenol) is another nonopioid pain medicine that helps reduce fevers, relieves mild to moderate pain, and strengthens the effects of opioid pain medication. It is often combined with opioid pain medication into a single pill in the form of acetaminophen-oxycodone (Percocet) and acetaminophen-hydrocodone (Vicodin). If you take one of these

Be sure to ask your doctor if you should be taking nonsteroidal anti-inflammatory medications if you have a history of gastric ulcers or chronic kidney disease. Nonsteroidal anti-inflammatory medications have wonderful anti-inflammatory properties; however, these same properties can decrease blood flow to the kidneys, and therefore patients with kidney issues should not take these medications. Also, these medications can cause gastrointestinal irritation or ulcers. Nonsteroidal anti-inflammatory medications should be taken with a meal to lessen the gastrointestinal side effects. If you develop stomach cramping or pains while taking these medications, you should notify your doctor.

Acetaminophen and Tylenol are the same medication. Acetaminophen is the generic medication name, and Tylenol is the brand name. It is important to read your prescription labels for information regarding medication, dosage, and frequency. Many surgeons may prescribe combination medications, such as Percocet (acetaminophen-oxycodone) or Vicodin (acetaminophen-hydrocodone), which have an opioid and acetaminophen in a single pill form. Therefore, you should not take extra acetaminophen in addition to combination medications that contain acetaminophen. Do not take more medication than prescribed.

combined medications, you should not take additional Tylenol. A general limit for acetaminophen is 3,000 mg in a 24-hour period. Overdoses of acetaminophen can affect your liver function and cause liver failure.

Diet

It is normal to have a loss of appetite for several days to a week after your surgery. This is often due to a combination of pain, medication side effects, and lack of mobility. You should be sure to drink plenty of fluids and stay well hydrated. It's important to eat well during your recovery in order to promote wound healing and recovery of muscle function and strength. You should avoid alcohol during your recovery and when taking opioid pain medication. If you are prescribed warfarin (Coumadin), then you should avoid certain food products that are rich in vitamin K. Coumadin works by blocking Vitamin K, which is essential for the production of coagulants in the liver. Eating foods that are high in Vitamin K will reverse the effects of warfarin. These foods include any green vegetables, such as kale, broccoli, cauliflower, Brussels sprouts, lettuce, cabbage, and green beans.

It is generally recommended to avoid smoking during the perioperative period, at least one to two months before and after surgery. People with diabetes should meticulously maintain a steady, safe blood glucose level.

Smoking increases your risk of infection by decreasing your wound healing potential. It is important to abstain from smoking cigarettes and cigars for at least a month before and after surgery. While nicotine patches also decrease blood flow and wound healing, they are still better than smoking while in the recovery period. If you are having issues with quitting smoking, please let your surgeon know. If you need support or help to quit smoking, you can call 1-800-QUIT-NOW or visit www.smokefree.gov /tools-tips/speak-expert.

Sleep

It can be difficult to get a good night's sleep after a total hip replacement. This is often due to sleeping more during the day as you recover as well as pain at night that may prevent you from sleeping. Pain is an important cause of difficulty sleeping, so be sure to take pain medicine prior to going to bed. It is important to realize that within two or three weeks, your activity level will increase as you strengthen your muscles through workouts and physical therapy, and therefore at the end of the day, you may have more pain than you did in the initial first few days after surgery. Ask your doctor or physical therapist what sleeping positions are allowed to help you get a good night's rest while also protecting your new hip replacement.

Leg Swelling

It is normal to have mild to moderate leg swelling for up to a year after your total hip replacement. To reduce leg swelling, keep your legs elevated (especially at night), ice them, and wear compression stockings when possible. Other exercises that can reduce leg swelling are ankle pumps and leg pumps, which contract your muscles and push fluid from your legs up toward your heart.

Although rare, one of the major possible complications in total hip replacement surgery is deep vein thrombosis (DVT), or the formation of a blood clot in the veins of your leg after surgery. Your orthopedic surgeon will prescribe a medication to prevent DVT, such as a scheduled aspirin regimen, warfarin, apixaban (Eliquis), rivaroxaban (Xarelto), or dabigatran (Pradaxa). Your orthopedic surgeon will determine the type and duration of DVT prophylaxis (prophylaxis means a measure to preserve health). Usually, medications are prescribed by your surgeon for a month after surgery, and daily aspirin might be continued in combination with another prescription medication. There is still a small risk of DVT, even when taking prophylactic medication and doing regular exercise. A more serious complication of DVT is a pulmonary embolism (PE). A PE occurs when a blood clot in the veins of your lower leg breaks free and travels to your lungs, resulting in blocked blood flow. PEs are a rare but dangerous complication that can be fatal, so their prevention is paramount.

Signs that you have deep vein thrombosis:

- Pain unrelated to your surgery in your leg
- Tenderness or redness at or below the knee
- Unexplained swelling of the thigh, calf, ankle, or foot

Signs of a pulmonary embolism:

- Sudden onset of shortness of breath or chest pain

Signs that you have a DVT are severe pain unrelated to your surgery in your leg, tenderness or redness at or below the knee, heat or warmth in the affected leg, or unexplained severe swelling of the thigh, calf, ankle, or foot. Signs of PE are sudden onset of shortness of breath or chest pain. If you have any of these symptoms, you should inform your orthopedic surgeon and go immediately to the emergency department for evaluation.

Diagnosis of a DVT can be done with a noninvasive vascular ultrasound, which looks at the veins in your leg and determines if a clot is present. If there is a question of PE, then often a chest computed tomography (CT) scan will be performed in order to evaluate your lungs.

If a blood clot or pulmonary embolism is found, it usually can be treated with a stronger blood thinner, such as warfarin, for a longer period of time, such as six months, to prevent an increase in size of the clot. Your body will naturally dissolve small clots. In the case of larger blood clots with critical blockages, your surgeon may recommend thrombolysis, whereby a catheter is inserted into your vein to either remove the clot or inject medicine directly at the clot to dissolve it.

Gastrointestinal Problems

It is normal to experience some constipation after a total hip replacement. It is important to take laxatives and stool softeners while taking opioid pain medication, because pain medicine slows down the movement of

your intestines, causing constipation. It is also important to get out of bed and walk as soon as possible. This
helps the bowel wake up and increases gut peristalsis
(movement of the gastrointestinal tract). If you are
severely nauseated, are not passing gas, or have severe
abdominal pain, it could be due to a paralysis of your
bowel, also known as an "ileus." In these rare cases, do
not force yourself to eat. Contact your surgeon or go to
the emergency department of your local hospital to be
evaluated.

Diarrhea is less common after orthopedic surgery.
If you develop persistent diarrhea or loose stools after
total hip replacement, you should report this to your
orthopedic surgeon and medical doctor. You may have
developed a gastrointestinal infection that requires further treatment.

Urinary Retention

Urinary retention after total hip replacement is
common due to immobility and side effects of hospital medications. Older male patients are at increased
risk of urinary retention due to an enlarged prostate. If
you are unable to urinate (void) after surgery, a urinary
catheter may be placed to relieve your discomfort. It
will be removed before you are discharged, and the vast
majority of patients will be able to urinate at this time.
If, however, you are still unable to void, then you may be
sent home with a urinary catheter to follow up with a

urologist in one week for evaluation and delayed catheter removal.

Fevers

Fevers are relatively common immediately after total hip replacement. By far the most common cause is atelectasis, which is a medical term for your lungs not being fully inflated, due to lying in bed and being immobile. It is important to practice deep breathing exercises and use a breathing device known as an incentive spirometer while in the hospital. Getting out of bed and walking also helps prevent this from happening. If you continue to not fully inflate your lungs, this puts you at risk of developing a postoperative lung infection (pneumonia). Other, less common causes of fever include pneumonia, urinary tract infection, DVT, PE, and surgical site infection.

It is helpful to have a digital thermometer at home. If you have a fever greater than 101°F, you should let your orthopedic surgeon know. You may need to be evaluated in the emergency department to rule out an infection.

Drains

Surgical drains are not commonly used after total hip replacement surgery. If you are sent home with a drain still in place, ask your surgeon for specific instructions on its management.

Moving into and out of Bed

Getting in and out of bed after your total hip replacement can be difficult. General considerations for getting in and out of bed after your total hip replacement are

- You will be most comfortable lying on your nonoperative leg.

- When lying on your side, put a regular bed pillow between your legs in order to prevent your legs from crossing.

- Keep your legs and knees shoulder-width apart when getting in and out of bed.

Remembering the above general rules and following the simple steps below will make it easier to get into and out of bed.

Getting into Bed

1. Sit on the side of the bed that will allow you to put your nonoperative leg onto the bed first.

2. Bring your nonoperative leg up on the bed first as you slide your bottom back onto the bed.

3. Finally, bring your operative leg up onto the bed. You may need someone to assist you with bringing your operative leg up onto the bed immediately following the surgery.

Getting out of Bed

1. Push yourself into a sitting position using your hands and elbows. You should exit the bed on the same side that you had your total hip replacement.

2. Continue to move your operative leg toward the edge of the bed. Use your nonoperative leg to help push yourself to the side.

3. Bring your bottom to the side of the bed and then slowly lower your operative leg to the floor.

4. Slide your nonoperative leg to the floor.

5. Use your arms and hands to steady yourself as you come up from a sitting position. It may be helpful to have your walker nearby to assist you in standing.

Bathing

In general, you will need assistance in getting in and out of a shower after your hip replacement. Often, surgeons will use waterproof dressings, and you may shower immediately postoperatively, but do not bathe until your operating surgeon instructs you to do so. You should not submerge your incision in water or tub bathe until your wound is fully healed, as this puts you at a higher risk of infection. Sometimes your surgeon will use a special waterproof dressing, which can be left in place for up to 14 days. You are allowed to shower with this dressing in place, but do not immerse your leg in a bath or pool until one month after your operation or per your surgeon's direction. Often, after the dressing is removed at two weeks, your surgeon will allow you to shower and let water run over the incision but instruct you not to scrub the incision. Certainly, do not scrub or pick at your incision.

Here are the steps to get into and out of a tub shower with a bench:

1. Ask a helper to set up a bench or a chair in the tub and make sure it is sturdy and does not move or slide.

2. Ask your helper to place any of your shower needs within reach, so you do not have to lean forward during the shower in order to maintain hip precautions as directed.

3. Stand with your back toward the bathtub with the bench behind you.

4. Ask your helper to hold the bench or chair steady while you lower yourself onto the tub bench or chair.

5. As you sit down, allow your operative leg to slide forward and slowly lower yourself down while maintaining control of your leg.

6. Once seated, lean your body and trunk back and have your assistant help you lift your operative leg over the edge of the bathtub. Remember to continue leaning back to maintain hip precautions.

Keep your leg straight, and do not cross your legs
or rotate your leg in and out when doing this. Have
your helper lower your operative leg slowly to the
floor.

7. In order to get out of the tub, have your helper lift
   your operative leg out of the tub and then lift your
   nonoperative leg out of the tub. Keep your feet
   straight and face forward. Have your feet flat on
   the floor before you stand. Use your helper and a
   walker for support when standing.

Here are the steps to get into and out of a shower
with a shower chair or bench:

1. Ask a helper to set up a bench or a chair in the
   shower and make sure it is sturdy and does not
   move or slide.

2. Stand with your back to the entrance to the
   shower and your back toward the shower chair.
   Your walker should be in front of you.

3. While using your walker, take a step back into the
   shower with your nonoperative leg and then bring
   your operative leg into the shower as well. Do not
   rotate or turn your legs, and keep your feet in front
   of you at all times.

4. Lower yourself onto the shower chair or bench
   while sliding your operative leg forward and leaning back. Remember to continue leaning back to
   maintain hip precautions.

5. When exiting the shower, use your walker to assist in pulling yourself up out of the shower chair. You'll need your helper to place the walker at the front of the shower after you're done showering. Do not use a towel rack or other unstable bars to pull yourself up or maintain balance.

6. Using the walker as support, slowly stand up from the shower chair. Step out of the shower with your operative leg, and then follow with your nonoperative leg while pushing down onto the walker with your hands. Regain your balance before exiting the bathroom.

Stitches and Staples

After your discharge, your orthopedic surgeon will give you specific instructions on wound care and dressing changes. There are many successful ways to achieve wound closure after total hip replacement. Some surgeons use staples or stitches, while others use self-dissolving subcutaneous sutures or skin glue. Staples or stitches are generally removed in the office two weeks after surgery. General guidelines are to keep the dressing clean and dry and change it as instructed by your surgeon. Your surgeon may use a waterproof dressing that should remain on for two weeks or until a follow-up visit. These dressings should not be removed unless instructed by your surgeon.

Your orthopedic surgeon will also tell you when it is safe to shower or bathe and get the incision wet. After showering, you should keep the incision clean and dry by patting the incision with a towel, and you should never rub the incision. If you have a waterproof dressing, then pat dry the top dressing with a towel. If the seal of the waterproof dressing is broken and water has leaked into the incision, then the waterproof dressing should be removed, the incision dried, and a new dressing applied. Call your surgeon if this occurs.

It is important not to tub bathe or submerge the incision in water until cleared by your surgeon, as this increases your risk of infection. It is also important to notify your surgeon if the wound appears red or if there is any fluid draining from the incision, as these may be signs of an infection.

Resuming Home Medications

Prior to discharge, talk with your surgical team about which medications you should take after leaving the hospital. Occasionally, antihypertensive medications should not be taken immediately after surgery due to low blood pressure caused by a combination of blood loss, anesthesia, and opioid pain medication. Immunomodulatory medications such as etanercept (Enbrel), adalimumab (Humira), and infliximab (Remicade) usually should not be taken for two weeks after surgery due to increased risk of wound complications and infections. If you are taking these immunomodulatory medications, consult with your rheumatologist prior to your surgery about when to stop and resume them.

Mobility

It is important to maintain mobility immediately after total hip replacement surgery. Movement helps prevent loss of muscle mass, constipation, blood clots (DVT/PE), and pneumonia and aids in overall recovery. The goal is to get you back to your day-to-day life as soon as possible. Initially, your physical therapist will have you walk with a walker.

After you have mastered the walker and are only using it for minimal support and balance, you will be transitioned to a cane. Consult your physical therapist prior to switching to a cane, which usually takes about one to three weeks after your total hip replacement. You should have your physical therapist with you when you're trying the cane for the first time.

Here are some guidelines for walking with a walker:

- Move the walker in front of you, so the back of the walker legs line up with your toes.

- Take a step forward with your operative leg to the walker, but do not step past the front of the walker.

- Then step forward with the other leg.

- Continue to repeat these steps.

Here are some guidelines for walking with a cane:

- Cane height should be adjusted so the top of the cane is at wrist level when you're standing with your arms at your side.

- Hold your cane with the hand opposite the leg that was operated on. The cane and the operative leg should work together.

- Move the cane forward about a step, take a step forward with your operative leg, and then step forward with your other leg.

- Continue to repeat these steps.

Resuming Activities of Daily Living

You should be able to resume most light activities of daily living, including preparing and cooking meals, dishwashing, and laundry, within the first three to six weeks following surgery. More rigorous activities of daily living, such as yard work and snow removal, may take several months to do without discomfort. When performing anything at home, please remember your hip precautions if you've been instructed to follow them. As you become more and more active at home, you may have increasing discomfort at night, which is common for several weeks after the surgery.

Always check with your surgeon about what activities you are allowed to do. In general, most surgeons recommend at least six to eight weeks before starting more vigorous activity with your hip, because this will allow the soft tissues to heal. Within the first six to eight weeks you're at a higher risk of dislocation or breaking your bones should you lose your balance and fall.

At about two to three months after your surgery, your surgeon may allow you to return to low-impact exercises such as golf, doubles tennis, walking, and cycling. A good exercise after total hip replacement is swimming. However, you should not start swimming until your physician has cleared you and your wound has fully healed. Most surgeons discourage repetitive, high-impact activities that include running and jumping. High-impact sports such as basketball, volleyball, soccer, and football are prohibited. Remember, the fewer miles you put on your hip, the longer it will last. The expected longevity of an implant is around 10 to 20 years, depending on activity level and your weight.

Most orthopedic surgeons recommend returning to driving at four to six weeks after surgery and sometimes sooner, if it's a left total hip replacement and if you drive an automatic transmission vehicle. There are some studies suggesting that reaction time for braking is decreased in the operative leg, and you should be aware of this when driving. You should not be taking opioid pain medication or other narcotics while driving.

When you can safely return to work depends on what type of work you do. More labor-intensive jobs, such as construction work, may take over three months of recovery. If you have a more sedentary job, like

It is important to ensure that you are a safe driver when getting behind the wheel. Do not drive impaired. Opioid pain medication, other narcotics, or mood-altering medications should not be used while driving. Studies have shown that reaction time for braking is affected by surgery, meaning that surgery on your hip will slow your ability to move your foot from the gas to the brake pedal. Before getting behind the wheel, you should discuss driving with your surgeon. Once you do start driving again, begin in an empty parking lot and ensure that you can move your foot from the gas to the brake pedal safely.

sitting at a desk or working on a computer, you may be able to return to work within four to six weeks, or potentially earlier, assuming that you are no longer taking narcotic pain medication.

Sexual Intercourse

It is usually safe to engage in sexual intercourse at four to six weeks after hip replacement surgery. This allows your hip time to heal and will prevent hip dislocation. General considerations are to prevent extremes of range of motion, twisting at the hip, and hyperextension of the hip (moving the leg backward). Usually, as long as the knees are kept apart from one another, dislocation risk is low. Begin with conservative, comfortable positions, and be gentle with your partner initially.

Rehabilitation

Functional Goals and Restrictions

Immediately after your total hip replacement, the goal is to resume walking and light activities of daily living. You will use a walker and continue physical therapy for strengthening and gait (walking) training. At 3 to 6 weeks, you should be able to resume most light activities, and you may walk with a walker or a cane, depending on how you progress. At 10 to 12 weeks, the expectation is that you will have returned to most, if not all, of your normal activities. It is important to note that vigorous activity or exercise should not begin until after 6 to 8 weeks from surgery, allowing the soft tissues and incisions to heal. Soon after surgery, you are at an increased risk of hip dislocation. Remember your hip precautions, which depend on the surgical approach used for your total hip replacement.

Exercises Done Lying Down

The following exercises can help strengthen your muscles and progress quickly through your recovery. Your physical therapist will give you many other exercises that you may continue to do at home. All of these exercises help strengthen the muscles of your leg and around your hip and aid in your recovery. The initial exercises can be done while lying in bed.

Ankle Pumps and Circles

Slowly push your foot up and down, pumping your ankle. You can then make circles with your ankle. Do this 5 times inward and 5 times outward. You should do these exercises 5 to 10 times in a row and repeat this 3 to 4 times per day.

Heel Slide

While lying flat, bend your knee on your operative leg and bring your heel toward your buttocks. Remember not to let your knee roll inward or outward and to keep your leg at the midline. You should do this 5 to 10 times in a row and repeat this 3 to 4 times per day.

Glute Set

Tighten your buttock muscles while lying flat and hold to a count of five seconds. You should do this 5 to 10 times in a row and repeat this 3 to 4 times a day.

Quadriceps Sets

Keep your leg straight while lying flat in bed, contract your thigh muscle (quadriceps), and try to make your knee straight. Hold this for 5 to 10 seconds. Repeat this exercise several times over a 10-minute period until your thigh feels tired.

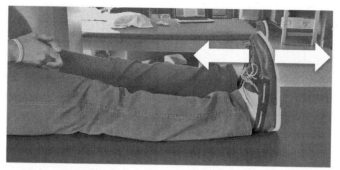

FIGURE 5.7. Ankle pumps

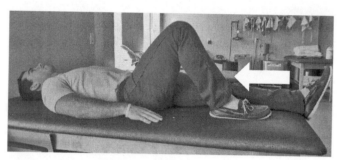

FIGURE 5.8. Bed-supported knee bends

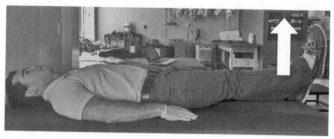

FIGURE 5.9. Straight leg raise

Exercises Done Standing Up

Once you are comfortable and have regained your strength, you may begin standing exercises. Make sure you're holding on to a walker while doing these standing exercises.

Standing Knee Raise

While standing and using a walker or stable chair for support, lift your operative leg toward your chest. Hold your knee up for 2 to 3 seconds and then push your leg down. You may do this 10 times a couple times a day. Do not lift your knee higher than your waist, maintaining hip precautions, and keep your leg straight at all times.

Standing Hip Abduction

You should not do this in the early postoperative period if you had a lateral approach surgery, as you need to give your abductor muscles time to heal. If you had a posterior or anterior approach surgery, you may do this exercise early on during your recovery. Make your hip, knee, and foot fully straight while holding on to a walker or stable chair for support. Keeping your body and knee straight, lift your leg out to the side and then slowly lower your leg back to your foot. Repeat this 10 times, a few times per day.

Standing Hip Extensions

You should not do this exercise if you have had an anterior approach surgery. While standing with your leg

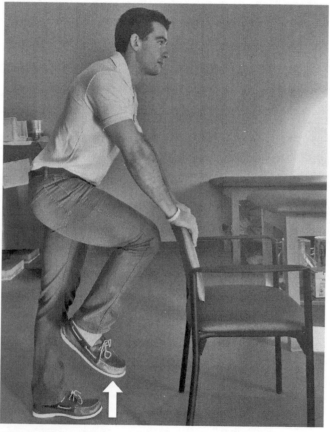

FIGURE 5.10. Standing knee raise

fully straight, hold on to a walker or stable chair and lift your leg backward slowly, keeping your back and knee straight. Hold for 2 to 3 seconds and then return your foot to the floor. Do this 10 times and repeat a couple times per day.

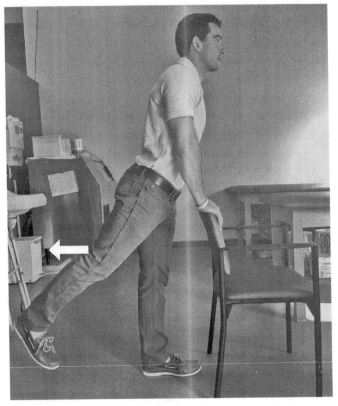

FIGURE 5.11. Standing hip extension

Suggested Timeline

If you have nonabsorbable sutures or staples, they will be removed at 10 to 14 days after surgery. You will be walking with a rolling walker or a cane and continue with physical therapy for strengthening and gait training. After 3 to 6 weeks, you will be able to resume most light activities and should have transitioned to a cane. At 10 to 12 weeks, the goal is for you to resume most normal activities you enjoyed preoperatively. Of course, every patient is an individual, and variations in progression through physical therapy can occur.

Follow-Up Surgeon Visits

First Follow-Up

Your orthopedic surgeon will set up a follow-up visit for two to four weeks after your surgery. You may visit your surgeon, their nurse practitioner, or their physician assistant at this time. This is to ensure that the incision is healing well and that there are no complications from the surgery. If you have staples or visible sutures, those will be removed at that time. You will continue to work with physical therapy. You will usually be walking with a walker or cane and may have outpatient physical therapy set up during this time if needed. Routine postoperative X-rays may be taken to document the position of your implants.

Subsequent Follow-Ups

Visits are usually scheduled for six to eight weeks and three to four months after surgery. Your orthopedic surgeon will check that you are continuing to progress as expected. At one year after surgery, there will typically be another visit to check on your progress, and X-rays usually are taken again at that time. Most orthopedic surgeons prefer to follow their patients annually, or every two or five years, for routine checkups and X-rays. Current research suggests that 80 to 90 percent of new total hip replacements will last 20 years.

Dental Treatment

As of 2016, a new "consensus" agreement now exists between the American Academy of Orthopedic Surgeons (AAOS) and the American Dental Association (ADA) regarding dental treatment after total hip replacement. For *all* people, daily brushing and flossing are recommended. People with healthy immune systems do not need antibiotics prior to dental work. People with a compromised immune system due to cancer chemotherapy, HIV/AIDS, or immune suppression medications, or those who have already experienced a joint infection after surgery, should have dental antibiotics prior to cleanings and treatments.

Check with your orthopedic surgeon regarding their recommendation prior to your dental visit and for their preference on duration of antibiotic premedication before dental cleanings.

Signs of Infection

If you ever develop increasing pain in your new hip replacement, you should be evaluated by an orthopedic surgeon. Warning signs of infection include persistent fever greater than 101°F, chills, redness, tenderness, drainage from the hip wound, and increasing pain. All of these warrant immediate evaluation. The risk of infection after total hip replacement done by an experienced surgeon using modern surgical techniques and implants is very low but not zero.

Points to Remember

- Your surgeon may recommend that you follow hip precautions to prevent hip dislocation. Make sure you understand your specific hip precautions and follow the precautions at all times.

- Opioid medications are important in the immediate postoperative period for pain control but should be taken less frequently over the first two weeks. The goal is to wean off the medication in the early postoperative period. Opioid pain medications, other narcotics, or mood-altering medications should not be used while driving.

- Some degree of constipation is normal after a total hip replacement. It is important to take laxatives and stool softeners while taking opioid pain medication.

- Mild to moderate leg swelling after surgery is common. To reduce leg swelling, keep your legs elevated and iced and wear compression stockings. Ankle pump and leg pump exercises also reduce swelling by contracting your muscles and pushing blood from your legs up toward your heart.

- Do not shower until your operating surgeon instructs you to do so. You should not submerge your incision in water or tub bathe until the wound is fully healed and you have been instructed to do so by your orthopedic surgeon, as this puts you at a higher risk of infection.

- If you have a sustained fever greater than 101°F, you should let your orthopedic surgeon know. You may need to be evaluated in the emergency department to rule out an infection (surgical site infection, urinary tract infection, or pneumonia) or blood clot.

- It is important to maintain mobility immediately after a total hip replacement surgery. The goal is to get you back to your day-to-day living as soon as possible.

- Daily exercises, as instructed by your physical therapist or home exercise program, are important to your recovery. Goals and milestones should be set with your surgeon and physical therapist. If you are having difficulty meeting these milestones, you should discuss with your surgeon specifically what is preventing you from reaching your therapy goals (sometimes pain control or apprehension). Your surgeon will closely monitor your progress and will have you come back for additional follow-up visits.

- If you ever have any questions or concerns, always check with your orthopedic surgeon.

What medications may I continue before surgery?

This is best answered in your preoperative appointment with your surgeon as well as your primary care provider. Some medications are essential to continue, while others can safely be stopped around surgery. Be sure to write down which to continue, which to stop, and which to take at a lower dose. Sometimes, a hospital pharmacist will also call you to discuss these concerns prior to your surgery.

What is chlorhexidine soap, and why do I have to scrub the site of my surgery with it?

Chlorhexidine soap has been shown to decrease the amount of bacteria living on our skin. Many centers recommend that patients shower and scrub their surgical site prior to their procedure to decrease the amount of bacteria at the site of surgery.

Why do I have bacteria on my skin?

Everyone has bacteria that normally live on their skin and cause no bad effects on their health. These bacteria can be harmful if they get inside your body, including through a cut or a joint replacement surgery. Therefore, surgeons and hospitals take every precaution possible to prevent these bacteria from affecting your surgery.

Should I go home or to a skilled nursing facility for rehabilitation after my surgery?

Most surgeons now feel that home is the safest place for you to recover after your surgery, but this is only true if you are able to care for yourself and have someone who can check on you periodically. In some cases, the safest place for recovery is in a nursing facility until you are strong and independent enough to care for yourself.

Why can't I eat or drink after midnight on the night before my surgery?

Not eating or drinking after midnight should prevent vomiting before, during, or after your surgery, which could result in aspiration, or vomit going into your lungs. Generally, it is believed that all the food and drink you have consumed will pass from your stomach to your intestines within eight hours. Small amounts of water that you drink with your needed medications are not a significant risk for vomiting around the time of surgery.

Why do I need a ride to the hospital?

You may be able to drive to the hospital, but while you are recovering after your surgery, not walking as well, and taking pain medications, it is not safe for you to drive. Therefore, someone has to drive you to and from the hospital to ensure that you are safe.

When can I drive after total hip replacement?

Most orthopedic surgeons allow their patients to drive four to six weeks after surgery and sometimes sooner in the case of a left total hip replacement or if you drive an automatic transmission vehicle. There are some studies suggesting that reaction time for braking is decreased in the leg that was operated on, and you should be aware of this when driving. You should not be under the influence of opioid pain medication or other narcotics while driving.

RESOURCES

Arthritis Foundation: www.arthritis.org

American Association of Hip and Knee Surgeons: www.aahks.org

American Academy of Orthopaedic Surgeons: www.orthoinfo.org

Tammi L. Shlotzhauer, MD. *Living with Rheumatoid Arthritis*, 3rd ed. Baltimore: Johns Hopkins University Press, 2014.

The bone of the hip socket is called the **acetabulum** and is physically connected to the pelvis bones.

Anesthesia provider refers either to an anesthesiologist (a medical doctor) or a certified registered nurse anesthetist (CRNA—a nurse who has undergone specialized training in anesthesia and is supervised by an anesthesiologist).

The **anterior approach** to hip surgery has the benefit of low dislocation rates without the need to detach any muscles or tendons, but it can have a higher risk of skin numbness adjacent to the incision. The patient lies on their back during the procedure.

Approach to the hip is the direction and path taken to get to the hip joint to safely perform a hip replacement. Each "approach" to the hip requires spreading between or splitting different muscles. Your surgeon will likely use the approach they are trained in and feel most comfortable using and feel is best for you.

Arthritis refers to the wear and tear of our joints over time, specifically causing damage to the normally smooth, slippery cartilage surfaces. There are three main types of arthritis: osteoarthritis (OA), inflammatory arthritis such as rheumatoid arthritis (RA), and post-traumatic arthritis.

Arthroscopy is a procedure in which the surgeon will make two to three small incisions in the front and side of your hip and use a camera to visualize the inside of your hip joint. Hip arthroscopy is rarely used in arthritic hips at the present time because studies have not shown that it helps hip arthritis. Hip arthroscopy is usually recommended for young athletes after a sports injury, before any arthritis has developed, to reduce or eliminate soft tissue deformities that may progress to arthritis or to fix tears of the labrum, which is the cartilage ring around the hip joint.

An **assistive device**, such as a cane or walker, may provide substantial symptom relief. A cane can help reduce the amount of pressure across the hip when you walk and should be used in the hand opposite the affected hip. Using a long-handled grabber to pick things up off the ground may help reduce some pain from bending. Assistive devices are used following surgery to lessen pressure on your new hip joint and help you balance.

Blood thinners are given after surgery to address blood clots. Examples of blood thinners are aspirin, warfarin (Coumadin), clopidogrel (Plavix), apixaban (Eliquis), rivaroxaban (Xarelto), and enoxaparin (Lovenox). Blood thinners that have been taken prior to surgery may be temporarily stopped or continued at a different dose.

BMI (body mass index) is a calculation of your weight divided by the square of your height (kg/m2). If your BMI is greater than 40, your surgeon may recommend a weight loss program for you before proceeding with any surgery.

Cartilage is the normally smooth, slippery covering of the joint. It is damaged by arthritis.

Case managers, also known as care coordinators or navigators, facilitate your discharge from the hospital. They help to set up at-home services, such as skilled nursing or physical therapy visits, and order devices such as walkers or canes. Case managers can also help facilitate your transfer to a nursing facility if that is where you are planning on going upon discharge.

A **catheter** may be used during surgery to allow you to urinate into a container during the procedure. This prevents your bladder from becoming too full and lets the medical team keep track of your body fluid status. After surgery, the catheter is often removed as soon as you are able to move to urinate comfortably.

Chlorhexidine soap is a special cleanser used to clean your skin. Some hospitals use chlorhexidine wipes. These help to reduce the number of bacteria living on your skin and therefore reduce the risk of surgical site infection.

A **"circulator" nurse** is someone who is not scrubbed in the surgery, who typically supervises and records events that go on in the OR. This person is responsible for getting any equipment that is needed during the procedure, opening sterile boxes, and generally facilitating your surgery.

A **contracture** means that muscles and bone anatomy have changed to the point that the hip joint is stuck in one position.

Cyclooxygenase-2 (COX-2) inhibitors are similar medications to nonsteroidal anti-inflamatory drugs (NSAIDs) but may have less severe GI side effects. Celecoxib (Celebrex) and meloxicam (Mobic, a partial COX-2 inhibitor) are commonly prescribed to reduce pain and inflammation. You should not take NSAIDs and COX-2 inhibitors at the same time because then you might overdose on these medications.

Deep vein thrombosis (DVT) refers to a clot that forms in the larger veins of the legs or pelvis and can lead to leg swelling and pain. A pulmonary embolism (PE) is when a blood clot travels and becomes lodged in the blood vessels of the lungs, which impairs oxygen delivery to the bloodstream and the body; a large PE can be fatal.

Disease-modifying anti-rheumatic drugs (DMARDs) such as methotrexate, sulfasalazine, and hydroxychloroquine are commonly used to treat rheumatoid arthritis. Other DMARDs such as etanercept (Enbrel) and adalimumab (Humira) work by reducing the body's immune response and are also commonly prescribed for these conditions.

A **fellow** is a doctor who has graduated from residency and been selected for a fellowship to subspecialize in a specific part of orthopedic surgery, such as total knee and hip replacements. In many centers, fellows are qualified to practice orthopedic surgery on their own and operate independently.

The **femur** is the thighbone. The top end of the femur forms the "ball" in the ball-and-socket joint that is the hip.

A **floor** is the generic term given to the ward or area of the hospital with patient rooms. This is where the majority of your hospital stay will take place.

General anesthesia means that you will be asleep during your surgery and a tube will be placed into your windpipe to assist in breathing during the procedure (you will not be aware of this!). Your breathing will be aided by a ventilator or a machine that delivers anesthetic gas and measures the size and rate of your breaths to ensure that you have enough oxygen during the procedure.

The **hip** is a ball-and-socket joint formed by two bones. The bone of the hip socket is called the acetabulum and is physically connected to the pelvis bones. The top end of the femur, or thighbone, forms the ball. To help the two surfaces glide by each other, both the acetabulum and femur are covered in smooth, slippery cartilage. The joint space also contains a lubricant called synovial fluid that helps the hip joint glide and allows the cartilage on the two bones to move smoothly on each other.

Hip arthritis refers specifically to the loss of cartilage within the hip joint. As the bearing surface wears, the movement is no longer as smooth, thus irritating the joint and surrounding tissues as well as making muscles work through abnormal mechanics. It ultimately leads to complete degradation of the joint, and often a total hip arthroplasty (or hip joint replacement) is needed to restore motion and relieve this joint pain.

Some surgeons will place patients on **"hip precautions"** after surgery to decrease the likelihood of a dislocation. Depending on the approach to the hip joint used during surgery, your surgeon may place you on anterior, lateral, or posterior hip precautions. These precautions limit the way you move your legs, hips, and back so as not to dislocate your new hip joint.

In a **hip replacement**, both the ball (femoral head) and the socket (acetabulum) of the hip joint are resurfaced. Worn-out cartilage is removed, and the bone is prepared for implant placement. A stem usually made of titanium is press-fit or cemented into the femur, and a prosthetic femoral head made of metal or ceramic is then placed on top of that stem. After surgery, the surface that you are walking and bearing weight on is a metal or ceramic ball on a plastic or ceramic socket liner. As with natural cartilage, there is very little friction between the two surfaces, which allows restored smooth motion and the greatest implant longevity possible, typically 10 to 20 years.

Impingement pathology is when parts of your hip structures hit or bump against one another during movement of your joint, leading to pain or limited motion. Impingement pathology may speed progression of arthritis. The two main types of hip impingement are cam and pincer.

Inflammatory arthropathies, such as rheumatoid arthritis (RA), are caused by autoimmune disorders that cause the body's own immune system to attack joints and cause them to deteriorate. Such disorders typically involve multiple joints. In addition to affecting the cartilage, autoimmune diseases cause overgrowth of the lining of the joint, the synovium, which contributes to additional pain and swelling. RA is a systemic disease that will typically involve the medical care of a rheumatologist, who will prescribe and manage powerful medications, in addition to surgical care from an orthopedist.

An **IV**, or intravenous line, is used to give medications and fluids directly into your bloodstream while you are asleep or unable to take medications by mouth. Often, an IV will be left in place while you are hospitalized, just in case some medication needs to be delivered quickly.

Labral tears are rips in the ring of cartilage that surrounds your hip joint. These tears can cause mechanical symptoms of clicking and popping felt in your hip joint.

The **lateral approach** to hip surgery, or the anterolateral approach, has a very good track record for stability; however, it requires the surgeon to detach and then repair tendons in the strong hip muscles called the abductors, which may result in postoperative weakness, a limp, or muscle problems. The patient lies on their side during the procedure.

Medical clearance is when your primary care doctor evaluates you and pronounces you fit for surgery. In some cases, your primary care doctor may recommend obtaining further testing or further consultation with another specialist prior to surgery. In some cases, your surgeon may recommend that you see a cardiologist (heart specialist), nephrologist (kidney specialist), or another specialist.

An **MRI (magnetic resonance imaging)** may be ordered
to see if something else around the hip may be causing
pain or dysfunction. MRIs use magnets to produce a
three-dimensional image. An MRI is not as good as an
X-ray at showing gross bone anatomy, but it provides
additional detail regarding surrounding tissues and
helps with a diagnosis of bursitis, tendinitis, or other
conditions.

Narcotics (opioids) are medications prescribed to
decrease pain in the immediate postop period and
are seldom prescribed for long-term pain relief from
arthritis. Narcotic medications, although effective for
pain relief, have many side potential effects including
nausea, vomiting, slowed breathing, constipation, and
sleep disturbance. In addition to these side effects,
narcotic medications can be extremely addictive;
therefore, they should be used with caution. Common
narcotic medications are oxycodone-acetaminophen
(Percocet), hydrocodone-acetaminophen (Vicodin),
oxycodone, and hydrocodone. Tramadol (Ultram) is a
synthetic, non-opioid-derived analgesic.

NPO stands for *nil per os,* meaning nothing by mouth.
This abbreviation means a patient is ordered not to
have anything to eat or drink.

NSAIDs (nonsteroidal anti-inflammatory drugs) are a
class of medications available over the counter that
include aspirin, ibuprofen (Motrin or Advil), and

naproxen (Aleve) and that help reduce pain and inflammation. It is important to take these medications with food, or as "enteric coated" tablets, as NSAIDs can upset the stomach and can lead to serious complications like bleeding ulcers if not monitored.

Osteoarthritis (OA) is the most common type of arthritis and is a degenerative process, which occurs slowly over time due to repetitive stress on the joint. OA can affect any joint and leads to erosion of the protective covering of the joint (cartilage), leading to roughening of the surface, increased friction, bone-on-bone contact, growth of new bone known as osteophytes or bone spurs, and even loose pieces of bone or tissue floating in the joint, making pain worse or causing mechanical locking, clicking, or catching. OA typically affects patients aged 40 and older. However, certain people are genetically predisposed to OA and can develop it at an earlier age.

The **PACU**, or postanesthesia care unit, is where patients recover immediately following their surgery before going to their hospital room.

Pain management refers to the regimen of pain-relieving drugs you will receive and your instructions for how often, and for how long, to take them. Your orthopedic surgeon will prescribe you a multimodal pain regimen prior to leaving the hospital; this often includes a combination of acetaminophen (Tylenol), nonsteroidal anti-inflammatory drugs (NSAIDs), and opioid pain medication.

PAT, or preadmission testing, is standard before surgery in many hospitals. You will meet with anesthesia providers and nurses, have blood work done, and familiarize yourself with the hospital.

Physical therapy refers to specific exercises that can help increase your strength, range of motion, and flexibility. The goal of physical therapy is to strengthen the supporting muscles of the hip and leg to help reduce pain, stiffness, and swelling. A physical therapist can tailor a specific program for your individual needs. Once you are comfortable with your program you can do the exercises on your own at home. Preoperative physical therapy, or "prehab," may also improve available range of motion and strength in the affected leg, which may subsequently improve postoperative outcomes or expedite recovery if you do have surgery.

Physician Assistants (PAs) help physicians in both the operating room as well as the office and may assist in your surgery.

The **posterior approach** to hip surgery is a very common and safe approach for total hip replacement but may be associated with an increased risk of postoperative hip dislocation when compared to other approaches. The patient lies on their side during the procedure.

Post-traumatic arthritis occurs when an injury or trauma causes or accelerates damage to a joint due to fractured bone surfaces, disrupted blood supply, misalignment or fracture malunion, cartilage injury, orthopedic hardware, infection, or a host of other causes. Soft tissue injuries in the hip, such as **labral tears** due to **impingement pathology** as a child or adolescent, can also alter normal hip mechanics and contribute to post-traumatic arthritis.

A **power of attorney** is legal authorization for an individual whom someone selects to make all their medical decisions if they are unable to do so. This person is also known as a medical decision-making proxy.

Pulmonary toilet refers to taking deep breaths after surgery and clearing any mucus that may develop.

Rehabilitation refers to the work you will do to regain your strength, balance, and walking ability after hip surgery. It involves both physical therapy and using a walker and a cane.

A **resident** is a physician trainee who has already finished medical school and received his or her medical doctorate. This doctor has been selected into a residency program, such as orthopedic surgery, for an additional specialized five or six years of specific surgical training after medical school.

A **revision procedure** is a re-do operation to fix an existing joint replacement that is not functioning correctly. These often are surgeries of longer duration and have a more prolonged recovery period.

A **scrub nurse** or **scrub technician (tech)** is responsible for the sterility and management of surgical tools and implants. They keep the instruments clean, hand the surgeons the required instruments, and keep everything in the operating room sterile.

The **social history** helps the doctor with planning the recovery from surgery. An understanding of who lives with the patient and the makeup of the home can help predict whether the home will be a safe place to return to after leaving the hospital.

Soft tissues are non-bony tissues such as muscles, tendons, and ligaments.

Spinal anesthesia is a form of regional anesthesia whereby medication is introduced into the area around the spinal nerves in the back. This blocks nerve signals to and from the lower half of your body during an operation. You will not be able to move or feel your legs throughout the surgery and for several hours afterward. Spinal anesthesia is "awake" surgery, meaning that your level of consciousness is not affected and you may be able to hear members of the team talking and working during your procedure.

Steroids are powerful anti-inflammatory medications that can be injected directly into the affected joint. In some instances, corticosteroids are given orally, but local injection is thought to have a more beneficial effect when treating arthritic pain. Steroid injections reduce pain and inflammation in the joint but do not slow the progression of disease, nor does their effect last forever.

Vendor representatives ensure that the hospital is stocked with an adequate number of surgical components and instruments. They are well versed in their company's implants and are able to ensure the correct devices are being utilized by the nursing staff.

Vital signs are taken at many times before and after surgery. They include your heart rate, blood pressure, breathing rate, and temperature.

X-rays are the main test used to diagnosis hip arthritis. X-rays are painless images that use small doses of radiation to make a picture projection of your bones on a film plate.

ABOUT THE EDITORS AND CONTRIBUTORS

Editors

Adam E. M. Eltorai, PhD
Research Fellow & MD Candidate
The Warren Alpert Medical School of Brown
University

Alan H. Daniels, MD
Associate Professor
Chief, Adult Spinal Deformity Service
Department of Orthopedic Surgery
The Warren Alpert Medical School of Brown
University

Derek R. Jenkins, MD
Assistant Professor, Division of Adult Reconstructive
Surgery
Department of Orthopedic Surgery
The Warren Alpert Medical School of Brown
University

Lee E. Rubin, MD
Associate Professor
Chief, Division of Adult Reconstruction, Yale
University

Chief, Yale–New Haven Hospital Total Joint Replacement Program
Department of Orthopaedics & Rehabilitation
Yale University School of Medicine

Contributors

Roy K. Aaron, MD

Professor, Division of Adult Reconstructive Surgery
Department of Orthopedic Surgery
The Warren Alpert Medical School of Brown University

Valentin Antoci, Jr., MD, PhD

Assistant Professor, Division of Adult Reconstructive Surgery
Department of Orthopedic Surgery
The Warren Alpert Medical School of Brown University

Travis Blood, MD

Orthopedic Surgery Fellow
The Warren Alpert Medical School of Brown University

Eric Cohen, MD

Assistant Professor, Division of Adult Reconstructive Surgery
The Warren Alpert Medical School of Brown University

Matthew E. Deren, MD
Assistant Professor
University of Massachusetts Medical School

John Froehlich, MD, MBA
Adult Reconstruction Fellowship Director & Clinical
    Associate Professor
Department of Orthopedic Surgery
The Warren Alpert Medical School of Brown
    University

Dominic T. Kleinhenz, MD
Orthopedic Spine Surgery Fellow
Department of Orthopedic Surgery
The Warren Alpert Medical School of Brown
    University

Scott Ritterman, MD
Adult Reconstructive Surgeon
Premier Orthopaedics
Exton, PA

INDEX

cortisone injections. *See* steroid injections

Coumadin. *See* warfarin

COX-2 inhibitors, 28–29, 86

CPAP machine, 49

crutches, 70

CT, 91

cyclooxygenase-1 (COX-1), 85

cyclooxygenase-2 (COX-2), 85

cyclooxygenase-2 (COX-2) inhibitors, 28–29, 86

dabigatran (Pradaxa), 90

DEA, 85

decision making, about hip replacement, 33–40

deep vein thrombosis (DVT), 37, 89–91; diagnosis of, 91; as fever cause, 93; prophylaxis for, 76–78, 90, 100; signs of, 90, 91; treatment for, 91

dental checkups/treatment, 13, 14, 111–12

dentures, 49–50, 51, 52, 58

diabetes, 13, 32, 88

diagnosis, of hip arthritis, 10–11; X-rays for, 3, 10–11, 19–21, 22

diarrhea, 92

diet, 27, 39, 46, 87–88

disease-modifying antirheumatic drugs (DMARDs), 28, 29–30

drains, surgical, 93

dressings, 95–96, 98, 99

driving, 50, 84, 102, 103, 112, 116, 117

Drug Enforcement Agency (DEA), 85

drug use, street, 18

DVT. *See* deep vein thrombosis

elective surgery, 23, 33, 36, 40

Eliquis. *See* apixaban

Enbrel. *See* etanercept

enoxaparin (Lovenox), 14, 76

etanercept (Enbrel), 30

exercise: for deep vein thrombosis prevention, 90; done lying down, 104–6; done standing up, 107–9; for leg swelling reduction, 89; low-impact, 25–26, 102; for rehabilitation, 104–9, 113; weight loss and, 39

falls, 42, 44, 70, 71, 102

family and friends: at the hospital, 53, 54–55; as support system, 17, 35–36, 40; visits from, 44, 66, 78

family history, 17

fasting, 41, 46, 48, 52, 53, 54, 79, 116

femoral head, 64

femur, 8, 9, 37, 64

fevers, 93, 112, 113

flare reaction, 33

fluid intake, 54, 74, 79, 87, 116

follow-up visits, 110–11

Food and Drug Administration (FDA), 32

friends. *See* family and friends